A Manual of Basic Microsurgical Techniques

This is a practical surgical manual providing a step-by-step guide to basic micro-surgical techniques for the reconstruction of small vessels, nerves and vas deferens. This also includes access to videos demonstrating core microsurgical techniques.

Incorporating 40 years of experience gained by the teachers of the microvascular course at Northwick Park, the techniques described in this manual have trained generations of surgeons. Fully illustrated and with a clear, succinct text, this manual will enable the reader to master basic skills quickly and confidently.

Microsurgery is not difficult, provided it is taught properly: There is no magic formula, but it must be learnt slowly, patiently and step by step. This valuable resource will be useful for surgeons in training and in practice and for research workers who are increasingly using microsurgical techniques in their experiments.

A Manual of Basic Microsurgical Techniques

Sandra Shurey

Sital Vara

Abdul Ahmed

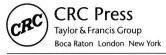

CRC Press is an imprint of the
Taylor & Francis Group, an **informa** business

First edition published 2024
by CRC Press
2385 NW Executive Center Drive, Suite 320, Boca Raton FL 33431

and by CRC Press
4 Park Square, Milton Park, Abingdon, Oxon, OX14 4RN

CRC Press is an imprint of Taylor & Francis Group, LLC

© 2024 Sandra Shurey, Sital Vara, Abdul Ahmed

ISBN: 9781032536743 (hbk)
ISBN: 9781032535760 (pbk)
ISBN: 9781003413080 (ebk)

DOI: 10.1201/9781003413080

Typeset in Calibri
by KnowledgeWorks Global Ltd.

Videos can be accessed via QR code on Video List page or the following link:

https://www.youtube.com/@microshuremicrosurgery483/videos

Contents

Video list   vi

Introduction   vii

Authors   ix

1   Equipment   1

2   Instruments   6

3   Stitch formation   13

4   Microsurgical training models   25

5   Animal model   28

6   Factors affecting anastomotic success   32

7   End-to-end arterial anastomosis   40

8   End-to-side anastomosis   56

9   Interpositional vein graft   67

10   Vessels under 1 mm   79

11   Anastomosis with single clamps   95

12   Continuous suturing techniques   104

13   End-to-side continuous suturing   115

14   Peripheral nerve repair   127

15   Rat vasovasostomy   135

16   Rat epididymovasostomy   142

17   Clinical practice   149

Index   157

Video list

Access to surgical videos demonstrating surgical techniques, together with step-by-step teaching modules to illustrate the techniques, is available via QR code.

https://www.youtube.com/@microshuremicrosurgery483/videos

Teaching Modules

Module 1	The operating microscope
Module 2	Instruments and suture
Module 3	Stitch formation and suture exercises
Module 4	Training models
Module 5	Factors affecting anastomotic success
Module 6	End-to-end arterial anastomosis
Module 7	End-to-end venous anastomosis
Module 8	End-to-side anastomosis
Module 9a	Interpositional discrepant vein graft
Module 9b	Interpositional vein graft
Module 10	Under 1 mm end-to-end anastomosis
Module 11	Under 1 mm end-to-side anastomosis
Module 12	Femoral artery to carotid loop
Module 13	End-to-end arterial and venous anastomosis with single clamps
Module 14	End-to-end anastomosis with continuous suturing
Module 15	Renal model with end-to-end continuous suturing
Module 16	Renal model with end-to-side continuous suturing
Module 17	Vasovasostomy
Module 18	Epididymovasostomy
Module 19	Nerve repair

Surgical Techniques

Video 0	Femoral vessel preparation
Video 1	End-to-end arterial microanastomosis
Video 2	End-to-end vein
Video 3	End-to-side anastomosis
Video 4	Discrepant vein graft
Video 5	Epigastric vein graft
Video 6	Nerve anastomosis
Video 7	Groin flap on the epigastric pedicle
Video 8	Groin flap end-to-side anastomosis
Video 9	1 mm arterial anastomosis utilising single clamps
Video 10	2 mm venous anastomosis utilising single clamps
Video 11	Artery anastomosis utilising continuous suturing
Video 12	Vein anastomosis with continuous suturing
Video 13	Carotid loop anastomosis
Video 14	Renal harvest
Video 15	End-to-end renal transplant with continuous suturing
Video 16	Renal transplant with end-to-side continuous suturing
Video 17	Vasovasostomy
Video 18	Vasoepididymostomy

Introduction

The object of this manual is to provide a step-by-step guide to basic microsurgical techniques for reconstruction of small vessels, nerves and vas deferens. Over the last 40 years we have absorbed, distilled and reworked information in light of experiments and research. The microvascular course at Northwick Park/Griffin Institute is the oldest in the country (began in 1979) and has been running for over 40 years, having trained generations of surgeons.

The need for microsurgical training in the UK was instigated by Prof. Colin Green, who was using microsurgical techniques in his experimental rabbit renal transplantation, and by three young, like-minded plastic surgeons – Michael Black, Gus McGrowther and Roy Saunders (all now professors!).

They realised that with the advent of clinical free flaps, the microsurgical aspect could not be acquired without some sort of formal training, and so the microvascular course was born.

I (Sandra Shurey) was there from the beginning and was mentored and encouraged by Prof. Green, who gave me the confidence to pursue a career in surgical research and microsurgery, and I owe everything since then to his wonderful guidance.

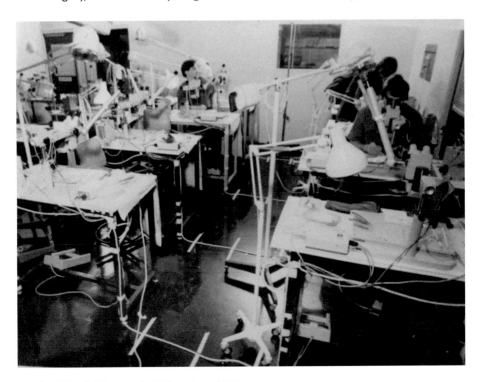

Northwick Park Microsurgical Workshop, 1979

We hope the manual will be useful for surgeons in training and practice and for research workers who are increasingly using microsurgical techniques in their experiments.

Some of the exercises would not be used clinically but are designed to enhance the microsurgical skills gained in a practice situation.

Microsurgery is *not* difficult, provided it is taught properly: There is no magic formula, but it must be learnt slowly, patiently and step by step.

In 1 week (~35 hours), it is possible for the average surgeon to master basic skills and, more importantly, prove to themselves that they are capable of doing them.

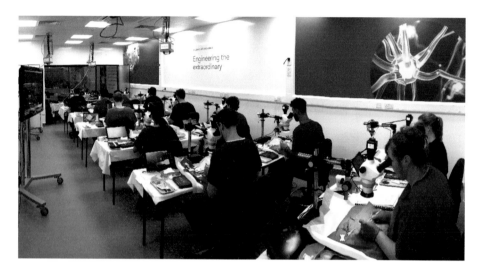

Northwick Park Microsurgical Workshop, 2023

Authors

Sandra Shurey, MPhil, is a Research Surgeon and the Co-Author of the training manual *Basic Microsurgical Techniques*. She has over 40 years of experience teaching microsurgery and to date has tutored over 4,000 surgeons from many differing specialties. She has had one manual, three book chapters and over 50 research papers published and has lectured internationally on microsurgical techniques. She has honed her microsurgical skills from a research background in organ transplantation (heart, lung, kidney, liver, pancreas and small bowel), also including free-flap, muscle transplantation, vasovasostomy, epididymovasostomy and nerve regeneration. She has also contributed to the assessment of microsurgical skills and to identifying the 'gold standard' for the running of microsurgical workshops throughout Europe. She also tutored microsurgery to medical MSc students from Imperial College, UCL and Queen Mary University and was nominated for an Honorary Lectureship at Queen Mary's. In 2016 when she retired, she started her own microsurgical training company: MicroShure Microsurgery and now teaches on a 1:1 basis from her home in Devon. She is still called upon for surgical research projects and still teaches and lectures on microsurgery at hospitals when requested.

Sital Vara, BSc, PGCert, is a Surgical Trainer and Research Surgeon and the current Director of the Northwick Park Microvascular course. Sital Vara has a background in surgical research, including wound-healing models, aneurysm repair and surgical implants. She has over 10 years of experience in small and large animal anaesthesia. She is an Honorary Lecturer for UCL and teaches undergraduate and postgraduate students basic surgical skills, including endoscopy, laparoscopy, microvascular surgery and robotic skills. Dr Vara has a passion for training and education and is involved in the organisation, management and continued development of various surgical training courses, including endovascular aneurysm repair courses, the London free-flap course and craniofacial trauma courses.

Abdul Ahmed, BDS, MFDSRCS, MBChB, MRCS, DO-HNS, PGCert, FRCS(OMFS), is a Consultant at OMFS/Head & Neck/Reconstructive/Robotic Surgeon. He is an Honorary Professor, Senior Clinical Lecturer at Queen Mary University of London and a Clinical Tutor at the Griffin Institute Surgical Training & Medical Research Charity. Bringing almost a decade of consultant experience in OMFS and head and neck surgery, Prof. Ahmed exhibits an innovative approach to his practice. He incorporates cutting-edge technologies, such as 3D planning, augmented reality (AR) and robotic surgery, into his work. With a notable repertoire, he has authored multiple textbooks and regularly imparts his knowledge through teaching engagements, including courses centered around microvascular surgery, reconstructive surgery and undergraduate/postgraduate training for several universities.

1 Equipment

Microscope

The cost of clinical operating microscopes is high, so the options for training are to buy a new basic model or to look around for second-hand microscopes.

Points to consider

- The depth of focus and breadth of field should be adequate even at high magnification.
- Some knowledge of the optical and illumination systems is valuable when selecting the most suitable microscope.

In our experience (working from a home or lab setup), there are now very good, cheap, reliable models to choose from.

Key recommendations

- Non-motorised, hand-operated on a bench stand
- Excellent optics and illumination
- 10× or 12.5× eyepieces
- Magnifications from 4× to 25×
- Working distance 175–300 cm

Optional

- Camera/video with live-streaming functions

Microscope mechanics

Optical system (Figure 1.1)

1. *Objective lenses*:
   a. These can be varied for focal length for working distance and brightness of the image.
   b. Those suitable for microsurgery are available in focal lengths ranging from 150 to 400 mm, but the standard is 200 mm (marked f = 200 mm).
   c. As the working distance increases, the amount of light reaching the operator is diminished.

DOI: 10.1201/9781003413080-1

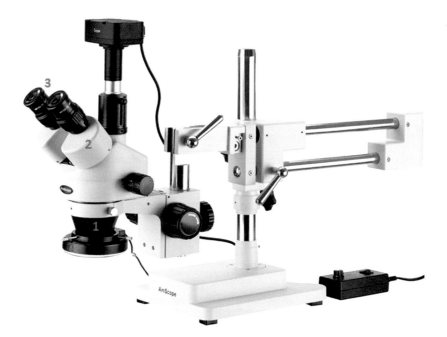

Figure 1.1 Microscope optical system.

2. *Tiltable binocular tube*: This is recommended, as it enables changes in microscope position during a surgical procedure for maximum comfort. It should also be adjustable so the eyepieces can be set to the correct interpupillary distance (IPD) for each individual.

3. *Eyepieces*: These are designed to magnify the intermediate image produced in the binocular tubes by the microscope objective. Eyepieces are described by their magnifying power.

4. *Illumination system*: It is also of prime importance. Several different types of light sources are available. The light system should produce minimal heat and be shock-proof, fail-safe and simple to operate.

   In use: The higher the magnification, the smaller the depth of focus and the less illumination is used.

Microscope care

Microscopes are easily damaged, and a few simple rules should be followed in their care:

● Never move mobile stands over rough surfaces on their own castors, and always remove and carry the microscope head separately.

● Clean the eyepiece and objective lenses with lens tissue every time the microscope is used.

● Clean the focus and zoom knobs after every session to prevent contamination with tissue.

- Always cover the whole microscope head in a plastic after use to prevent dust getting inside the instrument.
- Do not run the light sources at their highest intensity for longer than 5 minutes, as this reduces their life span dramatically.

Microscope setup

General hints for magnification (Figure 1.2)

- The lowest comfortable level of illumination should be used, as this is less fatiguing for the operator and ensures maximum life for the light source.
- The lowest level of magnification appropriate to each stage of the operation should be employed.
- High magnification (10× to 16×) is needed for preparing the ends of vessels and for passing the needle through the vessel wall.
- Low magnification (4× to 6×) is adequate for pulling the thread through and for vessel dissection.
- Intermediate magnification (6× to 10×) is used for actually tying the knots and for securing stay sutures to clamp cleats.

As microsurgery entails long hours spent in the same position, the surgeon's posture is critical. The height of the chair should be adjusted so that the operator is seated comfortably right up against the table's edge and with a straight, not curved, spine. If standing, it is paramount to keep the back straight.

Fatigue sets in rapidly if the neck is craned or the back hunched when accessing the eyepieces.

Adjusting the microscope

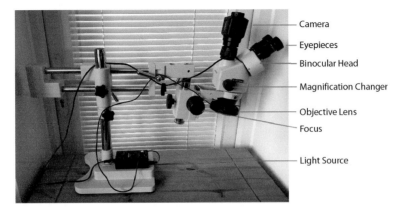

Figure 1.2 Microscope parts.

1. Position the microscope over the anastomotic area.
2. Switch on the light.
3. Rotate the engraved dioptre scale on each eyepiece to the zero position.
4. Set the microscope at its lowest magnification by operating the zoom knob or pedal.
5. Adjust the fine focus of the microscope so that it is in the centre of its travel (focus knob or pedal).
6. Move the 'body' of the microscope up and down until the anastomotic site is in focus, and tighten in position.
7. Keeping your eyes about 2 cm from the eyepieces, adjust the distance between the two eyepieces (IPD) until the two light images are superimposed on each other. Place your eyes close to the eyepieces and slowly adjust the distance until one image is perceived (the light will look a little brighter when the optimal image is attained).
8. With the microscope at its highest magnification (zoom knob or pedal), focus on the anastomotic area (focus knob or pedal).
9. Without altering the focus, change the magnification to its lowest setting (zoom knob or pedal).
10. If necessary, adjust each eyepiece setting to bring the anastomotic site into focus.
11. Make a note of the dioptre setting for each eye.

Surgical loupes

Loupes are often more convenient than the microscope for preliminary dissection and for anastomosis of vessels greater than 3 mm in diameter (**Figure 1.3**).

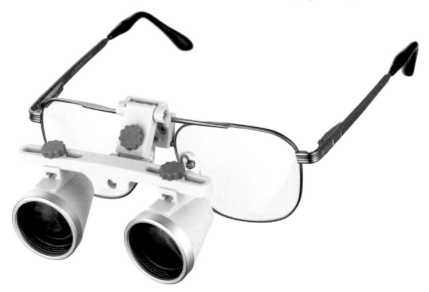

Figure 1.3 Surgical loupe.

A simple model with an elastic headband gives a magnification of 1.8×, whilst more sophisticated binocular loupes fitted to spectacles can provide up to 4× magnification without operator fatigue.

- Most surgeons choose 2.5×, as the microscope provides ~4× at its lowest setting.

- Some types of loupes have a wide field image, which can limit fatigue.

- When purchasing loupes, make sure they have a suitable working distance tailored to you.

An illuminated headband can be worn with loupes for extra clarity.

- In our experience, loupes with a higher magnification (8×) have too small a field of vision and depth of focus to be comfortable.

- Clinical loupes can be more expensive (>£1000) than a lab setup microscope, but there are cheaper options that may be useful for practice (~£177 Amscope).

- Some loupes are fully adjustable and can be adapted to each individual's need, but these can be more bulky and heavier to wear; others are tailored to the individual and are very lightweight, but they can only be worn by the person they are designed for and may need adjusting if the personal prescription changes.

2 Instruments

Purchase of a basic microsurgery set

It is a waste of time and money trying to skimp on instruments for the laboratory: If they are not good enough for use on patients, then they are not good enough to learn microsurgery in practice.

If possible, it is best for each surgeon to have their own set, which should then be looked after with care and never lent to anybody else (**Figure 2.1**).

Many variations on the basic microsurgical set are available from different manufacturers, but a few features to look for when making a purchase are common to all:

- They should have a satin finish to avoid glare under the microscope (black is good, if a bit more expensive!).

- Handles should be long enough to rest in the thenar web of the hand.

- Where instruments are spring-loaded, the closing tension should be sufficiently gentle to avoid fatigue.

Microsurgical instruments

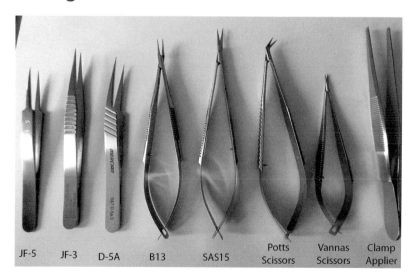

Figure 2.1 Microsurgery instruments.

DOI: 10.1201/9781003413080-2

Jeweller or Watchmaker forceps (Microsurgical forceps)

Microforceps

Nos. 3 and 5 are basic to any set and are used in the left hand for tying sutures and handling tissues.

Their tips must meet evenly over a length of 2 mm so that 10/0 and 11/0 nylon thread can be picked up easily without damage.

They can be either straight or curved.

Vessel dilator

- No. D-5a are microsurgical forceps modified at the tip so that they are rounded and polished.
- The closed tips can be inserted into the end of a divided vessel and then gently opened to provide counterpressure whilst suturing.
- We prefer to use these vessel dilators instead of the watchmaker forceps, as their offset design makes them easier to manipulate, they meet for a few millimetres at the tip to make suture tying much easier and their polished tip makes them less likely to cut through the suture material.

Needle holders

Purpose-designed models have spring-loaded handles, which can have a round or flat grip, and fine tips, which can be curved, angled or straight.

The tips should be fine enough both to hold the needle without distorting its designed curve *and* for tying knots.

Some of those on the market are fitted with ratchets for arming the needle, but in our experience, these should not be used because release of the lock is impossible to control and the needle can be easily damaged or lost.

Some surgeons prefer to use 45°-angled microsurgical forceps as needle holders because they are less expensive, have no hinges to corrode or snag the thread and they open and close easily.

Microscissors

Dissecting scissors

These should be spring-handled, and the curved blades can be short or long according to personal preference.

The blade tips should be rounded so that tissues adjacent to the vessels can be dissected without damaging them.

Adventitia scissors

These are identical to dissecting scissors, but the blades are straight.

Potts scissors

Their angled tips make them useful for performing arteriotomies and venomoties.

Vannas scissors

These are again spring-handled scissors with very sharp, pointed tips on fine, straight or curved blades.

They are used for removing the adventitia from vessels, cutting stitches and performing arteriotomies and venotomies in supramicrosurgery.

Vessel clamps

Acland clamps

Best for very small vessels, and the cleated frame is ideal for most microsurgical exercises (**Figures 2.2** and **2.3**).

Caution: The tiniest amount of blood or dirt in the joint can render them inefficient, and the jaws only meet for part of their length, so it is very easy for a vessel to partially slip and allow blood to leak from the cut end. In inexperienced hands, we would recommend single clamps proximally and distally in case of slippage.

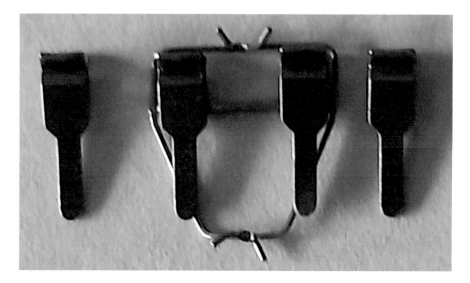

Figure 2.2 Acland clamps.

Other types of microclamps are available, but Acland clamps, in our opinion, seem to be the best. They are worth the expense, as they enable the surgeon to perform an anastomosis without help.

Tubal clamps

Winston modified Acland clamps for oviduct and vas deferens.

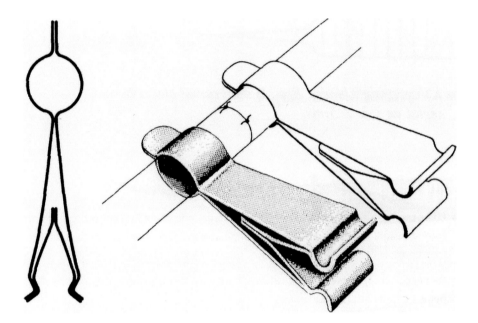

Figure 2.3 Tubal clamp.

Practice starter kit

- There are a vast variety of microinstruments available. A basic kit is all that is needed. This also saves time, as there will be less switching of instruments during an operation.

- A basic micropractice kit for home or lab use does not have to be expensive. Here is a suggested practice kit for chicken or rat models.

- An invaluable tool for irrigation is the Rycroft Air cannula. In our view, this is one of the most valuable microinstruments (**Figure 2.4**).

Care of instruments

Microsurgical instruments and clamps are delicate and easily damaged.

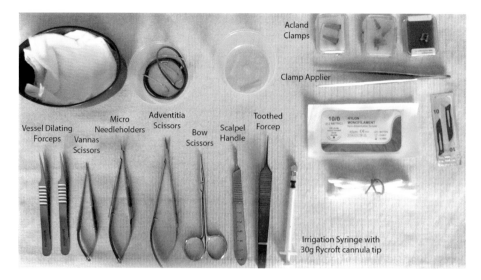

Figure 2.4 Basic practice setup.

In use

- Place them on a soft drape to prevent damage, and place in a set order each time they are used. It will then become second nature to pick them up without having to look up from the microscope.

- Damaged forceps may cut fine sutures; when not in immediate use, the tips should be protected with rubber tubing.

- Clamps should be placed in heparinised saline solution to prevent debris buildup and kept there whilst not in use.

- Repeatedly wash blood from the clamps and microsurgical instruments. Wipe with a damp gauze to remove debris as well as to help demagnetise the metal.

Cleaning

- A sign of a good surgeon is clean microinstruments at the end of the procedure.

- Dried blood on instruments can set hard enough to make a microforceps into a 'toothed' instrument.

- Additionally, flakes of dried blood can contaminate the vessel lumen.

- After use, the clamps and instruments should be cleaned with wet gauzes, then soaked in an enzymic solution for 45 minutes to dissolve any trapped clots.

- Rinse with a jet of water, taking care to get into the hinges, and place in an ultrasonic agitator for 3 minutes.

- Finally, they must be thoroughly dried and oiled before being stored away.

Microsurgical sutures

Suture materials

Monofilament polyamide (nylon) is noted for its smooth flow through tissue characteristics, its strength and its relatively inert behaviour in tissue. It knots well, and the black colour is clearly visible under the microscope (**Figure 2.5**).

Monofilament polypropylene (Prolene) and monofilament polyester.

Polypropylene sutures are inert, retain their strength in tissue well and the material is softer than nylon.

Advantages: Passes easily through delicate tissue because of their extremely smooth surface finish.

Disadvantages: Their light colour makes them more difficult to see under the microscope, and special care is needed when handling them to avoid damaging the material with surgical instruments.

All these materials are available in different sizes described as 8/0 (0.4 metric), 9/0 (0.3 metric) 10/0 (0.2 metric) and 11/0 (0.1 metric).

11/0 has a mean diameter of 18 µm, 10/0 of 25 µm, 9/0 of 35 µm and 8/0 of 45 µm.

Now available for supramicrosurgery: 12/0.

In our experience we much prefer nylon, as we have found that prolene does not knot particularly well, can be a little stiff and can be damaged during handling.

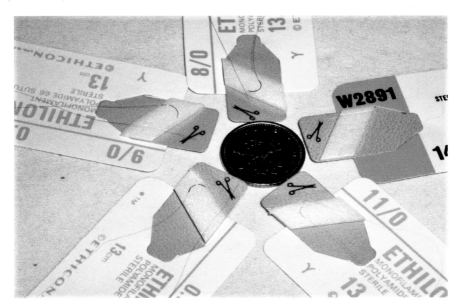

Figure 2.5 Microsurgical sutures.

Microsurgical needles

The monofilament material is swaged into one end of atraumatic 3/8 circle needles.

The following information is needed in selecting the best needle for the job:

- *Needle length*: This is the size of the needle in millimetres measured from point to butt around the outside curvature of the needle.

- *Needle profile*: This is invariably curved, but occasionally half-circle needles are used for end-to-side anastomosis.

- *Needle diameter*: This is measured in microns and is the critical measurement for microneedles. Diameters as fine as 30 microns are now manufactured.

- *Chord length*: This is the length in a straight line between the point and butt of the needle.

- *Cross section*: The vast majority of needles used in microsurgery have a tapered, atraumatic, round-bodied tip with a flattened rear end to make them easier to grip with needle holders. Micro-cutting needles are also available for nerve repair and tubal surgery.

- *Packaging*: Handling microsutures presents difficulties not found with normal suture dispensing, so all microneedles 100 microns in diameter and finer are packaged in a transparent envelope. The needles are inserted into a foam needle park, which can be removed from the sterile pack with the needle and suture, enabling the needle holder to be armed easily under the microscope. Non-sterile packs are now available.

3 Stitch formation

Handling microsurgical instruments

Practice card

The beginner should spend time on preliminary exercises on a rubber practice card (**Figure 3.1**) made from a rubber glove pinned to a cork board and using an 8/0 suture:

- Set the microscope for optimum use (see Chapter 1).

- Make sure your chair is adjusted to a comfortable height.

- Arrange your instruments on a draped tray in a set pattern so that they are easily reached without stretching.

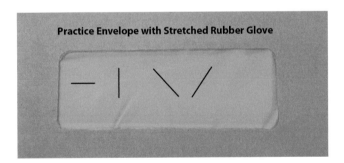

Figure 3.1 Practice envelope.

Hand position

Microsurgical instruments are handled like a pen, so the hands should be in the writing position (**Figure 3.2**):

- Resting on the hypothenar eminences and slightly supinated, knuckles outward.

- The elbows, wrists and ulnar border of the hands should be supported on the benchtop.

- Movements within the operating area should be restricted mainly to the fingertips.

DOI: 10.1201/9781003413080-3

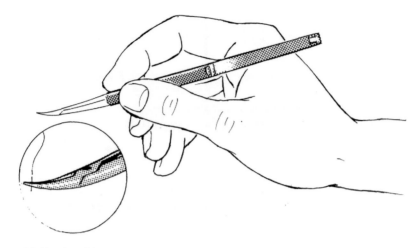

Figure 3.2 Hand position.

Use of microsurgical instruments

Under the microscope

● Practice rolling a needle holder in your dominant hand.

● Hold the forceps in the other.

● Bring the tips of the instruments to within 2 mm of each other in the same plane.

● Repeat until competent.

● Practice picking up instruments from the tray and bringing them into the microscope field.

● Never move instruments at the same time as you move your eyes from the microscopic to macroscopic field and vice-versa.

● Never move abruptly, but at a slow rhythmic pace.

● Move the instruments from the tray under direct vision into the general operative area.

● *Then* move them into the magnified area whilst looking through the microscope at low (4×) magnification.

Why?

● Microsurgical instruments are delicate and sharp and can easily damage blood vessels and tissues out of the operative field.

● Practice until these movements become automatic and instruments can be picked up and replaced without looking up from the microscope.

Needle handling

Picking up the needle

- Place the 8/0 suture in the centre of the magnified field (4×).

- Grasp the suture with the forceps about 5 mm from the needle; steadying against the rubber membrane, rotate the suture until the needle is pointing towards you.

- Grasp the needle with the needle holder (*always* with the convex curvature of the jaws facing downward) about a third away from the suture junction so that it sits about 2 mm from the tip of the needle-holder jaws.

- The needle should be at right angles to the needle-holder jaws and stable in this position (**Figure 3.3**).

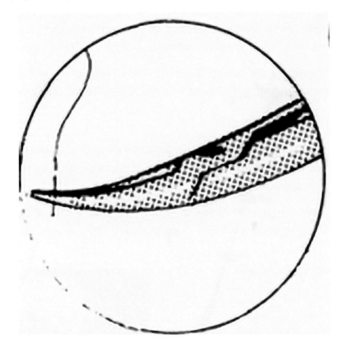

Figure 3.3 Needle position.

- Practice changing direction with the needle holder by flexion or extension of the wrist, and observe the needle point under the microscope as you roll the needle holder in your fingers.

- Repeat at a higher magnification (up to 10×) and establish for yourself the most comfortable magnification for this procedure.

- Only use as much magnification as needed. Remember the operating area is narrowed, the light is diminished and the focal length is much reduced at higher magnification.

Stitch formation

When learning stitch formation, it is essential to pay attention to detail. If the stitching is not executed properly, there is a high risk of anastomotic failure. It is extremely difficult to salvage a botched anastomosis, so it is *very* important to get it right first time, especially at the supramicrosurgical level. Time taken now to perfect stitches will save you many operative hours.

If a few simple rules are adhered to, the stitching becomes fluid and second-nature. Curiously, at the beginning of training, it is all about the suturing. When mastered, it is the least of your considerations in the micro-operative field.

The first exercise involves making 1 cm incisions with scissors into the rubber membrane: One horizontally, one vertically and two oblique. Five or six stitches are placed into these without moving the practice board. This ensures you can learn to anastomose at different angles, as you cannot always move your patient to the required position. We recommend the horizontal position to begin with, as this is the easiest position.

Imagine that the rubber is a delicate living tissue lined with intima which can be easily damaged and learn the same rigid rules now that you will need later in your patients.

Stitch formation: The procedure

- *Never* grasp the thickness of the 'tissue' between the jaws of microsurgical forceps, but evert it by placing the tips under the 'tissue' and allow the tips to spread about 1 mm apart (magnification 4×).

- Pass the needle through the 'tissue' at right angles[1] to the slightly everted surface at about 1.5× the tissue thickness from the edge using the dilator forceps as a counterpressure.

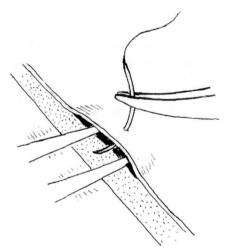 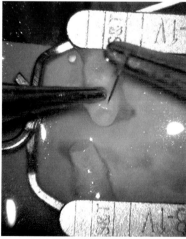

Figure 3.4 **Passing the needle.**

- With the microsurgical forceps now on the upper surface of the left side of the incision again as counterpressure, pass the needle through the left side at right angles to the wall and at the same distance from the edge. The suture should be passed from right to left at 90 degrees to the incision (**Figure 3.4**).

- Pick up the tip of the needle and pull it through, following the curvature of the needle. Do not attempt to pull it through in one straight movement, as you will make tears in the tissue.

Stitch formation: Knot tying

The knot instructions describe a true 'surgeon's knot', which in practice you will only need for stay sutures but are necessary in this case to hold the rubber material together.

Later, you will find that in most situations you only need to make a 'square' or 'reef knot' in which a single loop is used on each half-knot.[2]

If the knots have been made correctly, the cut ends should lie at 90 degrees to the incision and will not project downward into the incision or interfere with the next stitch.

The thread should be pulled through with the microsurgical forceps, again at 90 degrees to the incision, and guided by the jaws of the needle holders until only 5 mm of thread is left (**Figure 3.5**).

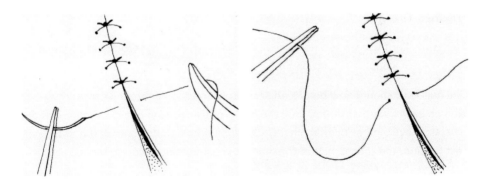

Figure 3.5 First stage of knot.

Figure 3.6 First loop of knot.

Place the needle on the periphery of the field and, with the microsurgical forceps, pick up the thread on the left of the incision about 1 cm from the suture holes (**Figure 3.6**).

Form a *double* loop around the tips of the needle holder by winding the thread clockwise around the jaws, which are kept stationary close to the incision (i.e., working in the same plane just above the tissue).

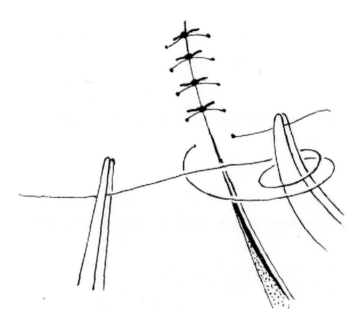

Figure 3.7 Second stage of double loop.

Pick up the short end with the needle-holder tips and pull with gentle tension whilst the double loops are allowed to fall from the jaws of the needle holder and thence over the short end of thread. Repeat this with knots at 0.5 mm intervals (**Figure 3.7**).

This is the knot used when performing the stay sutures that would be placed onto the cleats of a double Acland clamp.

The half-knot should now be placed accurately and then tightened carefully by tension on each length of thread until the edges of the incision come together without inversion, eversion or overlapping. Once the first half-knot is completed at the correct tension, the second half of the manoeuvre should not overtighten it.

Place the needle-holder tips over the middle of the knot, pass a single loop of thread over it in the reverse direction, pick up the short thread again and pull both threads in opposite directions in a straight line and at right angles to the incision.

For additional security, form another half-knot on top of and in the reverse direction to the previous half-knot (**Figure 3.8**).

Trim the short end of the thread first, then grasp the long thread still attached to its needle and cut that close to the knot. By pulling on the suture, you will pull the needle into view, ready to make the next stitch.

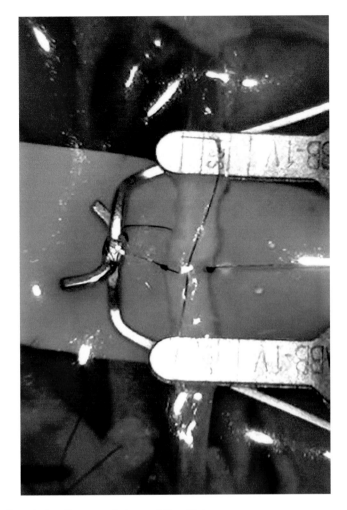

Figure 3.8 Completing the second phase of the stitch.

Rubber glove exercise

- Once the horizontal incision has been anastomosed, move on to the vertical incision.

- You will find that when starting to tie the stitch, your instruments will cross.

- Do not complete the tie, as there is a tendency to pull the suture more in one direction than the other, and this can cause a tear in the wall.

- Drop both ends of the suture, then pick up again with the instruments uncrossed and complete the stitch.

- Alternatively, if you throw the first loop of stitch around the microforceps and the second around the needle holder, this negates the crossover manoeuvre.

- When completing the oblique incisions, the stitches may not be at true right angles to the vessel edge, but as long as they are all in the same orientation, they will not interfere with each other.

- Depending on whether you are right- or left-handed, one of the oblique incisions will be more challenging.

- Resist the urge to stitch backwards, as you will not gain a full-thickness stitch.

- Instead, angle your hand around to achieve a forward stitch.

Simulated vessel exercise

Triangulation or 120-degree technique

The idea of this is to place the first two stay sutures at 120° and then apply horizontal tension. This flattens and stabilises the anterior wall whilst the posterior 240° falls away from the anterior. This helps to prevent catching the posterior wall when suturing the anterior and makes the anastomosis much easier to perform (**Figure 3.9**).

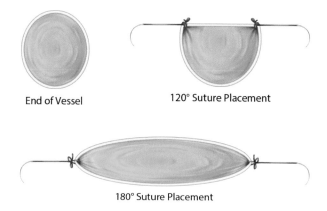

End of Vessel   120° Suture Placement

180° Suture Placement

Figure 3.9 Triangulation technique.

If the first two stay sutures are inserted at 180° and tension is applied, the two vessel walls 'sandwich' and the posterior wall can easily be caught in the anterior stitch (**Figure 3.9**).

Simulated vessel exercise

For this exercise, a 4 cm length of 1 cm diameter Paul's Penrose drain tubing is pinned out on a cork board and cut in half. 6/0 Prolene is used here, as the tube has a thick wall. Keep magnification low (4×).

Place two stay sutures 120° apart, one at 2 o'clock and the other at 10 o'clock, and leave a long thread to each so that these can be used to place horizontal tension on the anastomoses.

Put each stay under tension by trapping the thread between the head of a mapping pin and the cork board, thus keeping the upper wall of the divided tubing under lateral tension (**Figures 3.10** and **3.11**).

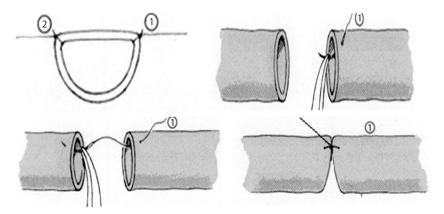

Figure 3.10 Placement of first stay suture stitch.

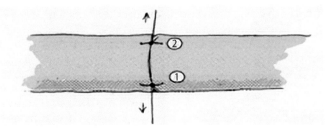

Figure 3.11 Placement of second stay suture stitch.

Anterior wall

On the anterior wall place another stay suture (#3) midway between the two previous stay sutures, leaving one end long (**Figure 3.12**).

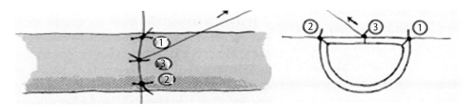

Figure 3.12 Placement of third stitch.

Fill in each segment between the stay and the traction sutures with sutures 0.5 mm apart, starting laterally nearest to the stay sutures and working toward the middle (#4 and #5) (**Figure 3.13**).

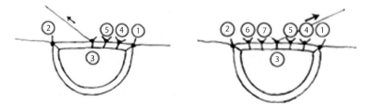

Figure 3.13 Placement of further anterior stitches.

Always add extra sutures from the stay suture toward the midpoint. This ensures that no unseen loose pockets of tissue can form next to the corner stay suture.

Release the stay sutures and turn the partially joined tubing over so that the unjoined posterior walls are now uppermost. Again, pin out the stay sutures.

Posterior wall

Use stay sutures throughout the anastomosis due to the 'vessel' tension. Because the vessel wall on this side is wider (through 240°), it is best to insert three traction sutures equidistant from each other, thus dividing the back wall into four segments. These are then sutured, working from the lateral stay sutures in towards the middle (**Figure 3.14**).

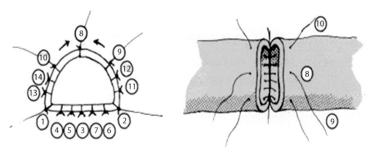

Figure 3.14 Placement of posterior stitches.

Repeat this exercise two or three times.

Cut the tubing longitudinally to reveal the internal wall and examine the sutures.

Assessment of suture lines

Be aware that simulated vessels are neither arteries nor veins. Suture spacing differs for both.

Arteries: One needle thickness between stitches to prevent bleeding

Veins: Two needle thicknesses between stitches to allow the vessel to dilate to maximum size on reperfusion

The sutures should be examined carefully on both the rubber card and simulated aorta to learn from any errors.

Make a critical assessment of your own stitching, looking for the following faults:

- Stitches too tight
- Stitches too loose so that a loop of suture intrudes into the lumen
- Too many or too few stitches
- Suture holes not equidistant from the edge so that the bite is not equal
- Uneven spacing between sutures
- Inversion or eversion of tissue edges
- Edges of tissue overlapping and heaped up on each other
- Stitch caught through both anterior and posterior walls

The perfect stitch

The perfect stitch should lie flat and straight so that the stitch ends are not raised.

Raised ends can infiltrate the lumen or interfere with subsequent stitch placement.

Stitches placed sideways interfere with visualising the next suture space and can also become entangled in the next suture placement (**Figure 3.15**).

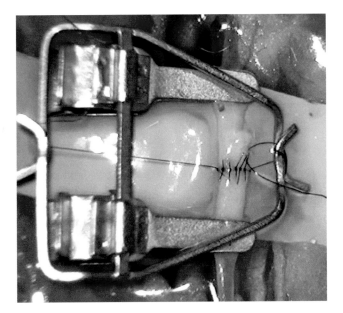

Figure 3.15 Perfect stitch placement.

For small vessels, use 4× magnification for preparation, then ~10× to place a stitch, then back to 4× to tie the stitch.

Take an adequate bite size for the type of vessel – remember 1.5× the thickness of the vessel wall.

When inserting the first two stay sutures, take the bites individually so as not to tear the lumen on the proximal side (**Figure 3.16**).

Once these are in, most stitches can be taken through both sides at once (**Figure 3.17**).

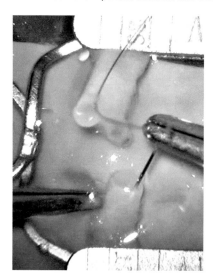 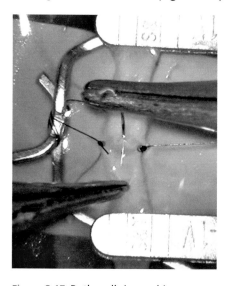

Figure 3.16 Individual wall bites.　　　　　Figure 3.17 Both walls in one bite.

Remember, always orientate the stitch to 90° of the anastomosis.

When forming a stitch, always place the needle holder in the middle of the stitch and form the stitch by pulling each loop down from opposite directions (failure to do so results in a build-up of loops that will not lie flat or tighten the stitch properly).

When tying, do not overtighten; just bring the vessel edges together.

When cutting ends:

● Cut the short end first (the needle is attached to the longer end so it is easy to recover).

● When cutting, cut both ends separately. Lifting both together results in the knot being raised and this can cause tears in fragile vessels.

● Always bring scissors in from the side so both ends can be seen before cutting the stitch.

Notes

1 The needle penetration angle will differ according to the thickness of the vessel wall. Thicker vessels will need the needle at a more vertical angle than a very thin-walled vessel.
2 Thicker-walled vessels may need another throw or two.

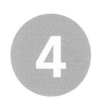

4 Microsurgical training models

Many models can be used for microsurgical training, and large funds are not needed. Though more expensive options are available for those with deep pockets, we have started with the cheaper options suitable for a home or lab setup.

Firstly, for stitch formation, a plastic bag, gauze swabs or background material can be utilised (use an 8/0 at 4× magnification).

Our favoured choice for beginners is a glove stapled to a card within an envelope.

This material is stretchy and more akin to a simulated vessel. The card can also be turned over for stitch inspection.

More expensive commercial versions are available from some surgical suppliers.

Once suturing on a flat surface at low (4×) magnification is mastered, then the next exercise is learning how to use the microscope to focus in and out at different depths of field.

A cork embedded with sewing needles at different depths can be constructed. A suture is then passed through each of the eyes of the needles in a continuous pattern. Following this, a stitch can then be formed on each individual eye of the needles using an 8/0 suture.

Natural materials can also be used to mimic very delicate structures. Try young leaves and grapes. Make an incision and then suture with 10/0.

Simulated tubes

The next stage is to use tubular models to simulate a mock vessel using the triangulation technique – this is described earlier in Chapter 3.

Penrose drain tubing is a rubber tube ideal for simulated anastomosis. Available in varying widths, the 35 mm is ideal to start with. Use 6/0, as the tubing is quite thick.

Silastic tubing is soft and easily takes a suture. It is available in many different widths and is suitable for the novice microsurgeon (use 8/0 and 10/0). The finest tubes are suitable for practising at supramicrosurgery levels (10/0 and 11/0) (**Figure 4.1**).

DOI: 10.1201/9781003413080-4

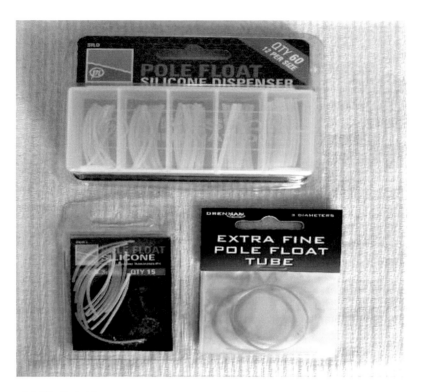

Figure 4.1 Silastic tubing.

Silastic tubing can be attached to connectors so that on completion of the anastomosis, leakage can be tested for (**Figure 4.2**).

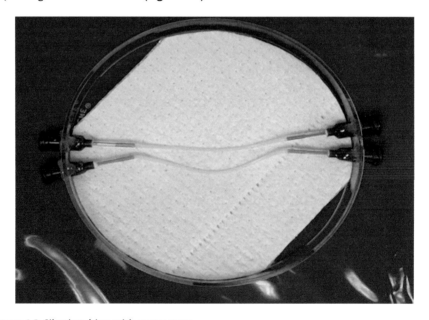

Figure 4.2 Silastic tubing with connectors.

Biological models

Japanese noodles are very fine and fragile but good models for practising supramicrosurgery (use 11/0).

Some students like to use earthworms, as they have a more 'vascular-like' structure for practice (use 8/0). Cryopreserved rat aortas are excellent models (use 10/0), as are umbilical cords if available.

The following models provide some microsurgical dissection skills as well as anastomotic practice. These larger models can include the pig or lamb heart. The coronary arteries can be freed and anastomosed (use 9/0). Pig or lamb spleens can also offer a myriad of vessels for anastomosis (use 9/0).

In our view, the best non-living model is the chicken thigh (a wing can also be used) (**Figure 4.3**). It involves some macrodissection and microdissection of the vessels and nerve (8/0 and 10/0) and can also be used to practise supramicrosurgical techniques on the side vessels (11/0).

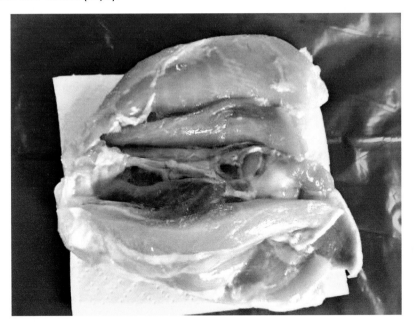

Figure 4.3 Chicken thigh.

Living model

The ultimate practice model is the living rat, as it provides immediate feedback on the quality of the vessel preparation and anastomoses and can also be used as a viable model for supramicrosurgery if the epigastric vessels are utilised.

Rat and chicken vessel dissection is explained in Chapter 7.

5 Animal model

General hints

In the United Kingdom, the Animals Scientific Procedures Act 1986 expressly forbids the use of living animals for acquisition of microsurgical skills unless a project licence and personal licence are first obtained from the Home Office. Initially, some suturing skills can, and should be, mastered on synthetic materials, on the chicken thigh or wing model or on isolated tissues such as cryopreserved rat aorta. The choice of these alternatives will depend on the availability of material and the level of technical expertise present in the laboratory. To get circulatory feedback, basic training must inevitably be completed in animals.

As the animals have to be fully anaesthetised for long periods before they are euthanised on completion of the operation, it is imperative that they are healthy before starting. If rats are used, it is best to select animals weighing 350–450 g, where their femoral arteries are about 1 mm in external diameter and the rats are still young enough to be reasonably free of chronic respiratory disease and are not obese. Ordinary, outbred (e.g. Sprague-Dawley) rats are suitable. Any rats with obvious symptoms of respiratory distress such as wheezing or sneezing should be avoided.

Anaesthetic management

It is only possible here to provide a few simple guidelines. In general, it is better to use injectable agents for these long microsurgical procedures, thus avoiding the hazard of operator exposure to inhalational agents. For long operations, it is best practice to ensure a source of heat to maintain body temperature, maintenance of fluid and analgesia.

Rats

Various combinations of injectable drugs can be used to anaesthetise rats. We favour urethane, which allows a prolonged anaesthesia, as rats can be anesthetised for up to 8 hours on the day of a course. Rats should be weighed prior to anaesthesia to ensure the correct dosage is administered.

The most important point is to find an anaesthetic regimen which works quickly and for the duration of the practice session, without the animal suffering any stress or pain. The anaesthetic procedure should be carried out by a licenced or suitably experienced person. The animal should survive the length of the practice session and

DOI: 10.1201/9781003413080-5

be terminated at the end of the session via an appropriate method. In the United Kingdom, this is called a schedule 1 method.

Short-acting anaesthesia

i. Ketamine at 60 mg/kg intramuscular (IM) with pentobarbitone at 20 mg/kg intra-peritoneal (IP) produces light surgical anaesthesia in 10–15 minutes, and lasts for 30–60 minutes

ii. Ketamine-acepromazine (premixed 15:1.0 mg/kg IP) produces light surgical anaesthesia in 10–15 minutes, and lasts for 60–120 minutes

Long-acting anaesthesia: Urethane with xylazine

Urethane requires preparation: 30 g of urethane crystals should be mixed with 100 mL of deionised water. All crystals should be dissolved, and the solution should be clear. Store at room temperature.

Urethane should be administered at 1.4 g/kg mixed with 20 mg/mL of xylazine IP, split into 3 doses. The first dose should be adminstered IP, leaving 1 mL remaining in the syringe. After 15 minutes a second dose of 0.5 mL can be adminstered IP. The final 0.5 mL dose can be administered 10 minutes later. Surgical anaesthesia should last up to 8 hours. If required, a top-up of 0.1 mL of urethane *only* can be administered IP to increase the depth of anaesthesia. This is likely to be required approximately 4–5 hours after induction to maintain a sufficient depth of anaesthesia.

The analgesic carprofen should be administered subcutaneously (SC) at 5 mg/kg with a 25-gauge needle. This lasts 24 hours, and no further doses are required.

To maintain fluid levels, 5 mL of normal saline (0.9% sodium chloride solution for injection) can be injected SC. If required, another 5 mL dose can be administered.

IM injections are made with a 10 mm × 25-gauge needle into the belly of the hind limb muscles or over the shoulders.

IP injections can be administered without the help of an assistant. The rat should be held firmly on its side, wrapped in a small, folded drape, with only its legs and lower abdomen exposed. Using a 25-gauge needle, the injection should be made in the lower right or left quadrant of the abdomen to avoid damage to other abdominal organs.

Anaesthetic depth is assessed on the respiratory rate and response to pinching the tail, interdigital web and ears. The latter is most sensitive in rats, and loss of reflex activity is a good index of full surgical anaesthesia.

Rats should be monitored constantly. Every half-hour, a full check should be carried out. This should include checking:

● Pain response from pinching the tail tip, ears or interdigital web

● Heart rate

- Respiration rate
- Any irregularities in breathing such as raspiness or wheezing
- Presence of a blink reflex

Rabbits

The main problem encountered during long periods of anaesthesia in rabbits is respiratory depression. It is therefore important to supply oxygen via a close-fitting face mask or an endotracheal tube (3.5 mm uncuffed paediatric tubes are ideal).

In the absence of inhalational anaesthetic equipment, the safest injectable agents in rabbits are xylazine at 7 mg/kg, followed 5 minutes later by ketamine at 20 mg/kg IM. This produces light surgical anaesthesia in 10–15 minutes. This will last for 30–60 minutes. To extend the period of anaesthesia, 15 mg/kg of ketamine *only* IM can be administered every 30–60 minutes as needed.

Having induced anaesthesia using xylazine and ketamine, long periods of anaesthesia can also be maintained using inhalational anaesthetic agents: 1–2% isoflurane with 1 L/min of oxygen via a mask or endotracheal tube should be sufficient to maintain anaesthesia for 3–4 hours.

Operating site preparation

It is far better to clip the hair from the operating site with the finest grade of clipper head (Oster 40®) rather than attempt to shave it. Loose hair should then be removed with a small handheld vacuum cleaner. For the exercises described later, it is worth clipping a wide area, including the lower abdomen, hind legs and scrotum (if males are utilised).

Rats are then laid out in the supine position on the operating board with the hind legs taped close to the board. The forelimbs should not be taped, as this will make thoracic excursions difficult and increase the likelihood of respiratory failure. The head and neck should be slightly flexed and not stretched straight, as this will diminish airway patency.

List of useful pharmacological agents

Anticoagulant: Heparin sodium supplied at a concentration of 1,000 IU/mL is useful both in the whole animal and diluted at 1,000 IU in 1,000 mL of isotonic 0.9% saline for irrigating vessels and the immediate operative site. In rats, approximately 100 IU/100 g body weight provides adequate anticoagulation.

Vasodilating agent: Lidocaine (2% solution) is useful in rats applied undiluted directly to the vessels and allowed at least 5 minutes to relieve spasm.

Respiratory stimulant: Doxapram (Dopram® 20 mg/mL) is a direct stimulant of the central respiratory centre and is effective in rats at 1.5 mg/kg IP to reverse respiratory depression.

Euthanasia

Rats should be terminated via an intracardiac (IC) injection of sodium pentobarbital at 0.6 mL/kg. Secondary confirmation of death can be achieved by cutting the femoral vessels (exsanguination) or cervical dislocation.

In rabbits, an overdose of sodium pentobarbital can be administered via an ear vein (3–5 mL). Secondary confirmation of death can be achieved by cutting the femoral vessels (exsanguination) or onset of rigor mortis.

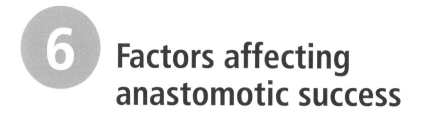

6 Factors affecting anastomotic success

Gentle dissection

This requires adequate gentle dissection of vessels. However good your anastomotic skills are, the vessels will not flow if damaged during the preparation stage.

Failure of patency in small blood vessels after anastomosis is caused by:

- Faults in microsurgical technique

- Alterations in the laminar flow of blood

- A tendency to coagulation and thrombosis after operation due to release of coagulation factors

- Spasm of the vessel musculature

- Or a combination of these

Poor surgical technique is undoubtedly the most important and is the most susceptible to improvement.

Microsurgical technique faults

The divided ends of vessels must *never be* grasped within the jaws of microsurgical forceps. Only grip the vessel by lifting gently from underneath or by grasping the adventitia.

- Gentle handling of the vessels is of prime importance, as the intima is very susceptible to damage. Try to avoid vessel spasm

- Traumatic placement of sutures, tearing of needle holes and multiple punctures are likely to trigger platelet aggregation

- Non–full-thickness needle penetration

- Uneven gaps or bites
  The correct bite and tension are indicated by a small suture loop whose diameter is roughly equal to the wall thickness and which is visible from the inside of the vessel.

- Inversion or eversion of the vessel edges leading to vessel narrowing

DOI: 10.1201/9781003413080-6

- *Tension*: Too much or too little

  Too much tension, which cannot be reduced within a double-approximator clamp, will cause stenosis of the vessel and tearing at the suture holes.

  If the whole anastomosis is put under longitudinal tension, either because the natural elasticity of a divided artery has allowed too big a gap to form or the vessels have been traumatised and need resection, then it is preferable to bridge the gap with an interpositional vein graft.

- Suturing the front and back wall together, thus constricting the lumen

  This is best avoided by using the triangulation technique described in Chapter 3. Keeping the walls widely separated whilst sutures are placed, repeated irrigation of the divided ends of the vessels and making a careful inspection of the lumen before tying the final sutures can help avoid this.

- Non-removal of adventitia

  In the case of arteries, it is important to remove the loose adventitial tissue so that it is clear of the suture line and less likely to be dragged into the anastomosis.

  Tiny tags of adventitial tissue can be carried into the lumen, and these are sufficient to form a nidus for platelet aggregation.

- Kinking or longitudinal torsion will again alter laminar flow and predispose to loss of patency. It can be a problem clinically when positioning free flaps or replants (**Figure 6.1**).

- *Clumsy tests for patency*: This includes overusing the 'milk' technique (see Chapter 7), particularly on vessels below 1 mm.

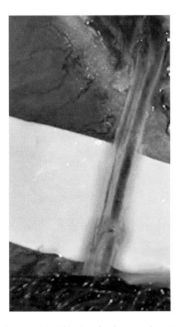 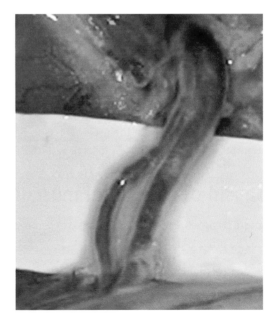

Figure 6.1 Effects of releasing longitudinal torsion.

Alterations in blood flow

Eddy currents and other forms of turbulent flow resulting from bends, kinks or gross distortion at the anastomotic site are likely to propagate thrombi downstream.

Turbulent flow can be observed most easily in an end-to-side anastomosis, but these cause surprisingly few problems so long as the suture line is not under tension and the incoming vessel is set at an angle between 60° and 45° with the direction of flow in the recipient vessel.

More important in any tissue transfer is poor flow or even complete stasis, particularly at the venous anastomosis. The latter will be at double risk if the arterial flow is inadequate because of partial patency, and hence flow through the microcirculation in the tissue is sluggish.

If veins are anastomosed such that they have a 'waist', then they will fail due to slow flow. Always anastomose veins at their maximum dilatation and this will not occur.

Most surgeons like to check the patency of the artery before proceeding to the venous anastomosis.

If a clamp is released and then applied again, it is important to remove any static blood by vigorous irrigation with heparinised saline before it starts to coagulate.

Release of coagulation factors

Any tissue or organ which has been compromised by hypoxia or ischaemia will build up toxic metabolites, including lactic acid, hydrogen ions, oxygen-derived free radicals and high concentrations of potassium.

These, together with thrombogenic factors such as bradykinins, serotonin and sensitised platelets, will be washed out of the tissue through the venous anastomosis once the clamps are released and further increase the risk of thrombogenesis.

Poor outflow is therefore the greatest risk in flaps and replants and has led to many attempts to improve results by local or systemic administration of inhibitors or leeches.

Spasm of the vessel musculature

Spasm (**Figure 6.2**) is almost inevitable at some stage in a microvascular procedure and may be provoked by:

● Surgical manipulation

● Exposure at the operative site to an unusually low ambient temperature

● Allowing the operative site to become dry

- Allowing blood or blood products in the operative field

- Abnormal pH and release of toxic factors from locally injured tissues

- It may also be provoked systemically via the sympathetic system by release of catecholamines

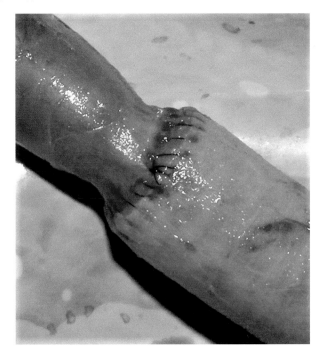

Figure 6.2 Spasm in a carotid artery to a synthetic graft (pig).

Prevention consists of careful dissection and constant irrigation of the immediate vicinity of the anastomosis.

Treatment is best achieved by applying a suitable topical vasodilator and allowing 10–15 minutes for the spasm to be relieved.

It is important to relieve spasm *before* attempting an anastomosis; it becomes much harder to space sutures evenly and the suture line may leak once it is relaxed.

Discrepancy in vessel size

There are various ways of coping with discrepancy in vessel size. The first solution is to do an end-to-side anastomosis, but if this is not possible, three other techniques are available:

- If the discrepancy is relatively minor, then it is possible to dilate the smaller vessel by gently inserting dilating forceps and spreading their tips, but there is a risk of damaging the endothelial intima.

- If the difference is greater, then the end of the smaller vessel can be transected on a 45° diagonal, thus providing a larger diameter edge for anastomosis (**Figure 6.3**).

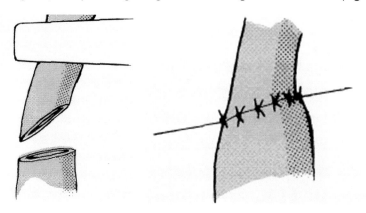

Figure 6.3 Forty-five-degree diagonal transection.

- Alternatively, the end of the small vessel can be incised longitudinally to create a 'fishtail', which can then be sutured to the larger vessel (**Figure 6.4**).

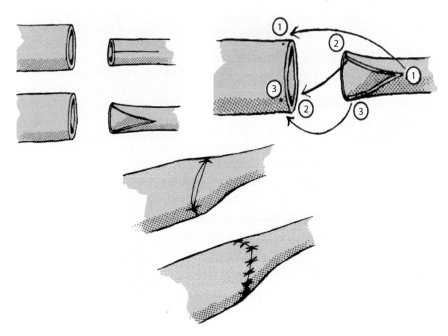

Figure 6.4 'Fishtail' of vessel.

In each of these methods, it is difficult to perform the simple triangulation technique, so great care must be taken not to suture the front wall of the vessel to the back. It is also very important to ensure that the vessels are under no tension, or the smaller vessel is likely to tear.

Similarly, you must ensure that the sutures are placed at the same relative position around the circumference of both vessels, or gaps will be left on insertion of the final sutures.

Summary of factors affecting anastomotic success:

- Rough handling

- Poor dissection technique

- Stitches too tight

- Stitches too loose so that a loop of suture intrudes into the lumen

- Too many or too few stitches

- Suture holes not equidistant from the edge so that the bite is not equal

- Uneven spacing between sutures

- Inversion or eversion of tissue edges

- Edges of tissue overlapping and heaped up on each other

- Stitch caught through both anterior and posterior walls

- Vessel stitch tears

- Tension on vessel

- Vessel spasm

- Discrepant size

When to repair or redo

Be 100% sure of your anastomosis. If you are only 99% sure and there is any doubt at all, then redo. This will save a lot of anguish later if you have a middle-of-the-night call for a failed flap.

If flow is compromised in any way:

- Narrowing at anastomosis

- Stitches caught through

- Stitch tears

- Uneven, tight or loose stitches

- Tension (graft if necessary)

Repair

- If a stitch has been misplaced, it is possible to carefully remove it and replace it, preferably before clamp removal.

- For general oozing, replace the proximal clamp and wait for a few seconds more, then recheck flow.

- For a pulsatile leak: Reapply clamps, find the gap, then flush all the blood out with heparinised saline before placing an extra stitch and then retesting.

- Trying to add an extra stitch to a bleeding vessel will result in a misplaced stitch; the defect will be hard to see due to blood flow, so reapply the clamps and flush.

- More importantly thrombus will be 'locked in' if the static blood is not removed, and anastomotic failure will ensue.

Any 'waist' present on a venous anastomosis will almost certainly lead to failure.

Always anastomose veins at full horizontal stretch (maximum dilatation), and this will be avoided.

Human factors affecting anastomotic success

Personal comfort

Standing for long periods can lead to bad backs and stiff necks. Make sure you stay as upright as possible and comfortable at the microscope. We have found that the mountain pose (taken from yoga) facilitates long periods of standing.

Mental efficiency

- Mental rehearsal and visualisation techniques have been used in sports, music, aviation and recently, in training in laparoscopic surgery with successful results.

- The concept is to mentally rehearse the anastomosis in significant detail so that the surgeon can visualise each step vividly in their mind (including detailed imagery cues) prior to undertaking the task itself (**Figure 6.5**).

> **A Randomised Control Trial Exploring the Effect of Enforcement of Mental Rehearsal and Cognitive Visualisation on Microsurgery Skills**
>
> Priyanka Chadha, MBBS, BSc(Hons), MSc, MRCS2 Nadine Hachach-Haram, BSc(Hons), MBBS, MRCS1 Sandra Shurey MPhil 3, Pari-Naz Mohanna, FRCS(Plast)2

Figure 6.5 Mental rehearsal.

Don't panic

- When we start to panic, then fight, flight or freeze takes over and governs fear and anger. This emotional hijacking leads to strong emotions and makes us stupid.

- Panic and tremor set in and make the anastomosis doubly hard.

- Taking time to panic is time lost to set things right.

Coping mechanisms

Most surgeons are reluctant to let colleagues know that they are not coping or are panicking if the anastomosis is not going well. We have some suggestions to help you cope that can be done without anyone realising that you are suffering.

The adrenalin surge experienced during this is accompanied by sharpened (foveal) vision, a dry mouth and shallow breathing.

Mechanism 1

- To dampen the response, look away from the microscope. Go into peripheral vision – soften your focus, bring saliva into the mouth and take three slow deep breaths.

- You will find your anxiety will lessen and you can start to think more rationally.

Mechanism 2

- 7/11 Breathing: To dampen the adrenalin response, try to breathe in for a count of 1–7 then breathe out for a count of 1–11.

Mechanism 3

- *Drop-through technique*: This can be accessed again without anyone noticing.

  - Think of the emotion you are experiencing e.g., frustration.

  - Then think of the next feeling e.g., anger.

  - Carry on until you can no longer access any emotion – you will come to a void.

  - Think of the emotion under the void, and you will strangely find a positive emotion e.g., calm.

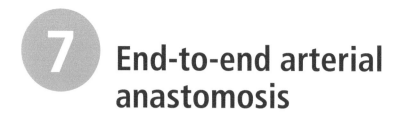

7   End-to-end arterial anastomosis

Vessel exposure

Chicken

The first incision is made ~1 cm below the bone to expose the next muscular layer. Below this is the vessel plane. Expose the vessels and nerve and dissect them free. Do not detach the vessels at either end or their stability will be lost (**Figure 7.1**).

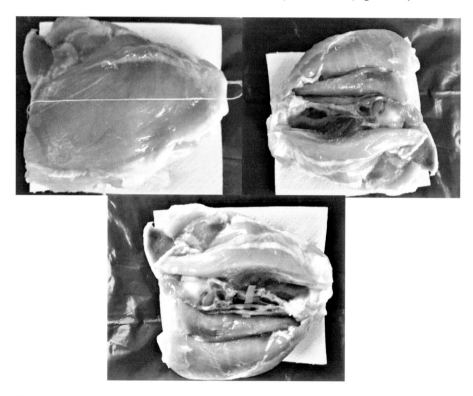

Figure 7.1 Chicken vessel exposure.

Rat

Place the anaesthetised rat on its back and tape out the hind legs in a slightly extended position. The femoral triangle is bounded proximally by the inguinal ligament.

The femoral vessels lie deep to a thick inguinal fat pad and are covered by a thin sheet of fascia (**Figure 7.2**).

DOI: 10.1201/9781003413080-7

The first stage of the dissection is to make a longitudinal incision from the inguinal ligament to just above the knee.

The fat pad should be picked up and incised at the distal end and raised by blunt dissection until the femoral artery and vein are revealed together with the nerve entering the leg through the femoral canal.

The fat pad should be retracted laterally to the left at the same time hooking a retractor over the abdominal musculature and inguinal ligament and retracting this medially.

The full length of artery and vein can then be visualised to the distal point of the femoral triangle.

The femoral vessels give off the superficial epigastric artery profunda femoris vessels, which dive deep into the underlying muscle.

The profunda femoris vessels are important in this dissection, as they have to be ligated and divided to leave a sufficient length of femoral vessel for the double-approximating clamp to be placed and turned over.

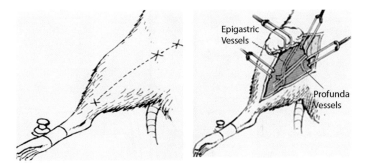

Figure 7.2 Rat femoral dissection.

Vessel dissection

As described in the rat; the chicken dissection is similar.

- Having exposed the whole of the femoral triangle, the next stage in the dissection is to separate the loose overlying fascia and then prepare the artery and vein.

- Under low magnification (4×), pick up the dense femoral sheath with your forceps, gripping the sheath well away from the vessels.

- Nick the sheath at its distal end with the blades of the dissecting scissors parallel with the surface and slide one blade into the nick and thence away from you along the sheath. The sheath is thus opened longitudinally for the full length of the femoral triangle.

- The artery can now be freed from the septum by gentle lateral and longitudinal teasing using No. D-5a vessel dilating forceps in each hand.

- Vessels should be picked up only by the loosely attached adventitial tissue or raised from underneath with the sides of the closed forceps tips.

- Longitudinal stress must be avoided to minimise the risk of constriction and spasm.

- Having freed the artery for its full length, it is time to ligate and divide the profunda femoris artery.

- Slide a No. D-5a forceps under the profunda femoris artery, raise it gently clear of the parent vessels and then it can be cauterised (**Figure 7.3**).

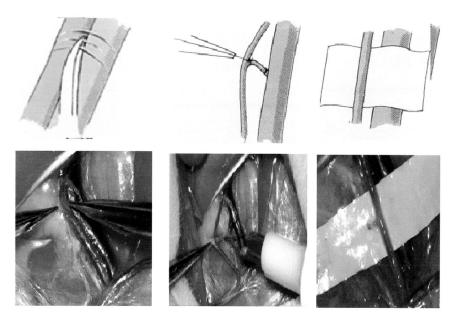

Figure 7.3 Dissection of the femoral artery.

- The vein can now be freed from the septum by gentle lateral and longitudinal teasing using No. D-5a vessel dilating forceps in each hand.

- Vessels should be picked up only by the loosely attached connective tissue or raised from underneath with the sides of the closed forceps tips.

- Longitudinal stress must be avoided to minimise the risk of constriction. Having freed the vein for its full length, it is time to ligate and divide the profunda femoris vein.

- Slide a No. D-5a forceps under the profunda femoris vein, raise it gently clear of the parent vessels and then doubly ligate. Using No. D-5a forceps, pass a 7/0 suture around the branch and tie off close to the femoral vein. Leave the ends of the suture long so that these can be pulled to one side.

- Gentle traction on the profunda femoris vein allows access for the second ligature to be placed before the vessel is divided between ligatures.

The profunda femoris vein should be divided between ties and not simply cauterised, as this can be insufficient to prevent bleeding; the vein must be dissected with extra care.

Scissors should definitely not be used, and the surrounding tissues should be teased *away* from the vein with No. D-5a forceps.

The veins are very thin walled, lack a substantial muscularis and are easily torn. They are best handled by the small pieces of fat adherent to them.

Finally, the whole field is irrigated with saline, and a piece of background material is slipped under the chosen vessel so that the two vessels are temporarily isolated from each other.

However good your anastomotic skills are, the vessels will not flow if damaged during the preparation stage (**Figure 7.4**).

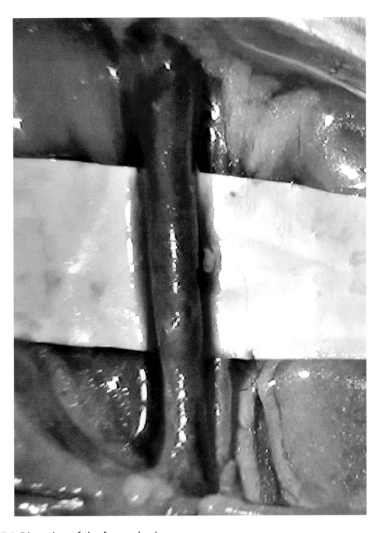

Figure 7.4 Dissection of the femoral vein.

Arterial anastomoses

The routine described here is for the Acland vessel approximating clamp (ABB-1), but this can be adapted to other types of double clamps on a slide bar.

The main point of having the two clips on a bar is to allow them to slide towards each other and thus ensure that the divided ends of the vessel are brought close together and are under no tension whatsoever whilst being anastomosed.

● Having rinsed the ABB-1 in heparinised saline, place it in the operating field viewed under low magnification, and slide the two clips as far apart on the bar as possible.

● Slide the whole frame over the background material and under the artery until just the clip tips project slightly beyond the vessel with the artery lying in a straight line over the two clips (**Figure 7.5**).

● With the clamp appliers, open first the proximal clip, grasp the artery by its adventitia and pull it longitudinally into the open clip before allowing it to close. Now open the distal clip, and again pull the artery longitudinally toward the centre of the frame, slide it into the clip and allow this to close (**Figure 7.6**).

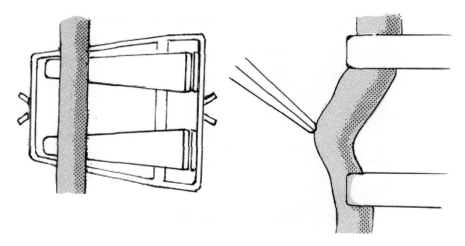

Figure 7.5 Clamp placement.   Figure 7.6 Arterial clamping.

This manoeuvre ensures a relaxed length of artery between each clip. Do not twist the vessel and ensure that it is held at the *tip* of the clip; clamping the vessel nearer the clamp bar will lead to vessel slippage when the clamp is pivoted.

● With the scissors at a right angle to the vessel wall, the artery should be transected halfway between the two clips with one decisive but controlled movement to achieve a clean cut through the full thickness of the vessel. The divided ends will retract immediately.

- Irrigate the vessel with heparinised saline using a 30-gauge Rycroft Air cannula attached to a 1 mL syringe.

- The clamps are now slid gently towards each other until the retracted vessel ends are close together. If ample arterial length has been included between the clamps, then they will only need to be pushed together a little, thus leaving plenty of room for the anastomosis without the clamps getting in the way when the needle is being passed (**Figure 7.7**).

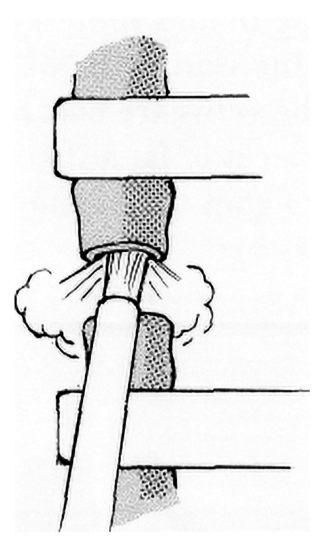

Figure 7.7 Irrigating the artery.

The chicken artery is non-viable, so it will not retract as much once transected, so just apply clamps without pulling too much excess artery between the clamps

- The femoral triangle should now be thoroughly irrigated until it is full of fluid and the divided ends of the vessel are floating freely. Only then is it possible to see the loose adventitial tissue properly. It is important to remove this for 1–2 mm from the anastomosis edge.

- The simplest method of doing this is to grasp the tissue with No. D-5a forceps and pull it gently over the vessel end until a cone or sleeve is formed. Amputate it cleanly in one snip at the level of the underlying stump. The remaining tissue will retract back, leaving the vessel with a clean end (**Figure 7.8**).

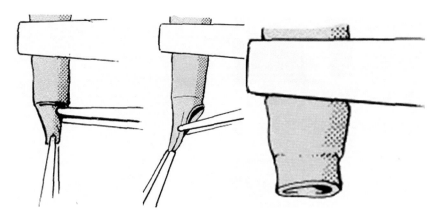

Figure 7.8 Removing arterial adventitia.

The chicken artery has very little adventitia, so do not overstrip.

The anastomosis is performed using the triangulation or 120° technique described previously in Chapter 3.

- The first stay suture is now placed at 2 o'clock around the circumference.

- Using ~10× magnification, place the closed tips of vessel-dilating (No. D-5a) forceps just inside the lumen of the proximal vessel and slightly open them or raise the vessel open by grasping the adventitia.

- Place the needle tip overhead and slide it back to a point of entry about 1.5× the thickness of the vessel wall from the edge.

- Pass the needle perpendicularly through the vessel wall so that it emerges between the forceps tips, acting as a counterpressor, and follows the curve of the needle until two-thirds of its length is through (**Figure 7.9**).

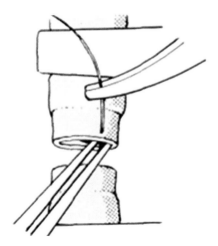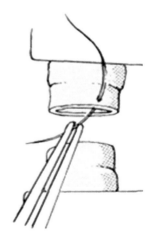

Figure 7.9 Needle placement.

- Transfer the needle holder to the lumen, grasp the needle about its midpoint and pull it through clear of the wall together with about 5 mm of suture. The adventitia of the distal vessel is now grasped with the forceps and is used as a counterpressor whilst the needle is passed perpendicularly from the vessel lumen.

- The holder grip is again transferred to the front segment of the needle, and the suture is slowly pulled through in one continuous movement, using the closed forceps to guide the suture through the proximal entry point in a straight line and so prevent it from tearing and enlarging the hole toward the edge of the vessel (**Figure 7.10**).

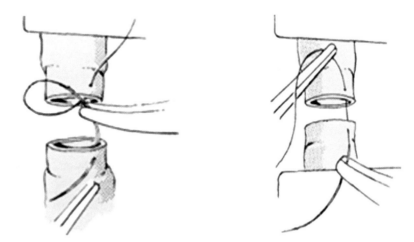

Figure 7.10 Needle placement through both arterial walls.

- Leave about 3–4 mm of suture projecting from the entry point. Alter the magnification to ~6× and lay the needle down near the edge of the visual field where it can be picked up.

- Grasp the long arm of the suture with the forceps about 1 cm from the exit point and form a double loop around the tip of the needle holders by winding the suture clockwise whilst keeping the holder tips stationary close to the vessel edges – this avoids the risk of pulling the whole suture through so that the entire procedure has to be started again (**Figure 7.11**).

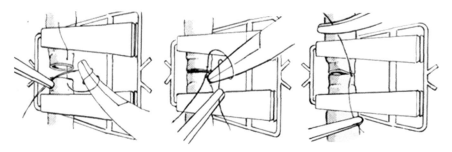

Figure 7.11 First throw of stay stitch.

- The short arm of the suture is now picked up in the holder jaws and pulled from top to bottom at the same time as the long arm still gripped by the forceps is carried over from bottom to top. The double throw must lie flat against the tissue at right angles to the suture line, just bringing the vessel edges together until they abut each other.

- To form the second part of the surgeon's knot, place the needle-holder tip over the middle of the existing half-knot, pass a single loop of suture over it in the reverse direction, pick up the short thread again and then pull both threads in opposite directions in a straight line and at right angles to the vessel edges (**Figure 7.11**).

- For additional security, place a third tie as a forehand loop. Trim only the short end of the suture.

- Using the forceps and needle holder, secure the stay suture in the cleat in a figure-of-eight, placing the stay under gentle traction.

- Place the second stay on the opposite side of the front wall 120° apart, and secure it to the other cleat with sufficient traction to stretch the anastomosis line laterally (**Figure 7.12**).

The front wall is now sutured using square or reef knots, which must lie flat against the anastomosis line. Under no circumstances must 'granny' knots be made, as the ends can easily project through the suture line and into the lumen. Each suture must penetrate the full thickness of the vessel wall, and the bite should be about 1.5× the vessel wall thickness.

For intermediate sutures, it is easier to pass the needle through both sides of the anastomosis in one movement without releasing the holder.

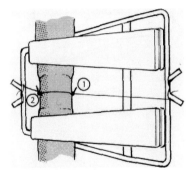

Figure 7.12 Completion of both stay stitches.

● First, place one suture (the holding suture) equidistant between the two stay sutures and leave one end long so that it can be grasped with forceps to raise and stabilise the vessel walls whilst intermediate sutures are placed.

● Turn the clamp over *before* tying this suture, taking great care that the cleats do not snag or puncture the adjacent vein, and make sure that you have not picked up the back wall. If all is well, return the clamp back again and complete the reef knot.

● The next suture is placed near the first stay suture, and thereafter they are placed at intervals approximately one needle diameter apart, working towards the middle. Always check the back wall before tying each suture to confirm the back wall has not been included in the stitch.

● The other quadrant of the front wall is completed in the same way.

The long uncut end of the middle suture has been used to steady the anastomosis for each of these sutures, thus avoiding all unnecessary handling of the media or intima; this technique is simpler and less damaging than picking up the adventitia with forceps (**Figure 7.13**).

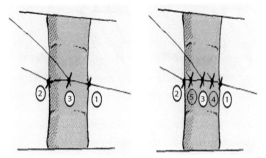

Figure 7.13 Anterior anastomosis.

● Having completed the anterior wall, irrigate and turn the approximating clamp 180° so the arterial posterior wall is revealed.

● Irrigate the lumen with heparinised saline.

- If necessary, nudge each clamp a little closer together to ensure that the suture line is not under tension (**Figure 7.14**).

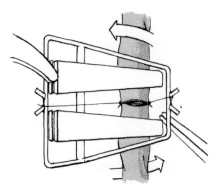

Figure 7.14 Releasing tension on the anastomoses.

- Place the first (holding) suture equidistant between the two stay sutures and, after tying a square knot, leave the top end uncut so that this can be grasped to pull the posterior wall away from the anterior and stabilise it whilst the needle is passed for the intermediate sutures. It is also used to apply slight lateral tension and to aid in even placement of the sutures (**Figure 7.15**).

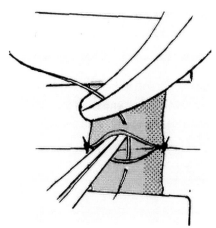

Figure 7.15 Placement of first posterior stitch.

- Complete the anastomosis as before, suturing each quadrant separately and working from the stay stitches towards the centre.

Completion of anastomosis

Arterial clamp removal

After irrigating the field, the clamp is now rotated back to its original position and the artery is checked to ensure that it is not adhered to the metal frame.

Divide the stay sutures close to the knots. The distal clip is opened first and the vessel slid out of the clip. Blood should immediately fill the vessel back to the proximal clip, having crossed the suture line (**Figure 7.16**).

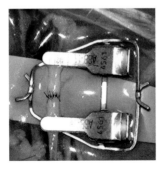 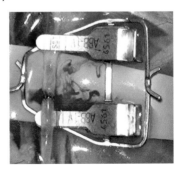

Figure 7.16 Distal clamp removal.

- Once the anastomosis has stopped oozing, open the proximal clip and slide out the artery.

- Under low magnification, apply gentle pressure over the suture line with microsurgical swabs and wait ~2 minutes for all bleeding to stop.

- Pulsatile bleeding must be considered a surgical failure, and another suture should be placed after reclamping and irrigating (**Figure 7.17**).

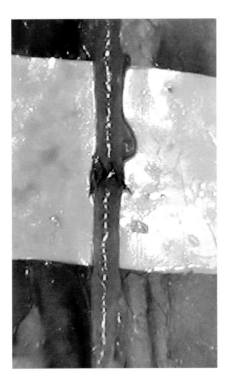

Figure 7.17 Clamp removal.

Assessment of arterial patency

It is difficult to check that the vessel is patent by simple observation because longitudinal pulsation can be transmitted distal to the anastomosis. However, if arterial tributaries are pulsating, then the anastomosed artery must be patent.

The 'Milking' test

The 'milking' test is a very reliable tool. The vessel is occluded just distal to the anastomosis with a pair of forceps, and the vessel is 'milked' for 3–4 mm distally with another pair of forceps, which are then used to occlude the vessel. This produces an empty length of vessel lying between the two occluding forceps. If the anastomosis is patent, the vessel should rapidly refill as soon as the proximal pair of forceps are released (**Figure 7.18**).

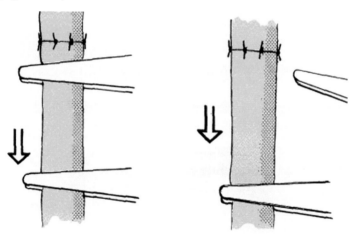

Figure 7.18 Milk test.

Surgeons like to play! Only perform the milking test *once*. Overtesting can ultimately damage the vessel.

One-way-up anastomosis

In some clinical circumstances, it is not possible to use a double-approximating clamp, in which case single clamps may be used and the stay sutures attached to the single clamps to hold the stay stitches under tension.

It may also be impossible to use the triangulation technique because the vessels cannot be turned over easily (due to lack of access or tension), so it may be necessary to suture the back wall first with one suture then gradually work around until the anastomosis is completed (**Figure 7.19**).

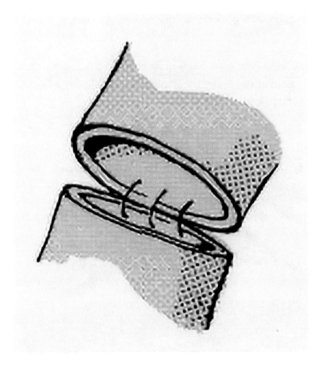

Figure 7.19 One-way-up anastomosis.

Venous anastomosis

This follows the stitch pattern of the artery, but there are a few differences in the venous preparation:

- Before clamping, ensure the vein is free of any connective tissue. Be careful not to overstrip. The venous wall should be shiny and smooth. If it becomes dull and 'woolly' then the wall has been compromised.

- Having rinsed the ABB-1 in heparinised saline, place it in the operating field viewed under low magnification, and slide the two clamps as far apart on the bar as possible.

- Then slide the whole frame over the background material and under the vein until just the clamp tips project slightly beyond the vessel with the vein lying in a straight line over the two clips.

- With the clamp appliers, open first the distal clip, grasp the vein, let it relax into position and then pull it longitudinally into the open clip before allowing it to close.

- Now open the proximal clip, let the vein relax into position and then pull longitudinally toward the centre of the frame; slide it into the clip and allow this to close.

- Clean off any loose tags of tissue and adherent fat, but do not attempt to remove adventitia, as this in not present in the vein.

Letting the vein relax into position before clamping prevents the vein from twisting during clamping.

Do not twist the vein (veins are very unforgiving if any twists or kinks occur), and ensure that it is held at the *tip* of the clip; clamping the vessel nearer the clamp bar will lead to vessel slippage when the clamp is pivoted.

● With the scissors at a right angle to the vessel wall, the vein should be transected halfway between the two clips with one decisive but controlled movement to achieve a clean cut through the full thickness of the vessel. The divided ends will retract immediately.

The chicken vein is non-viable, so it will not retract once transected, so just apply clamps without pulling excess vein between the clamps.

● Irrigate with heparinised saline and fold back each segment of vein over its clamp. This helps to display the lumen and orientate the vessel walls (**Figure 7.20**).

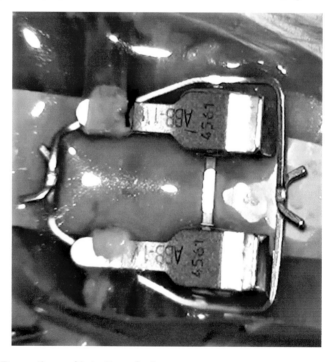

Figure 7.20 Transection and irrigation of vein.

● If necessary, slide the two clamps towards each other to approximate the vessel ends, but leave sufficient working space between them to perform the anastomosis in comfort.

● Fold the venous ends over the clamps to expose the lumen. The anterior wall is now resting on the clamp's surface.

- Submerge the veins in heparinised saline to prevent adherence of the vein walls, and place the 10/0 stay sutures at 10× magnification.

It is vital that maximum horizontal tension with the stay sutures be applied so that the vein is anastomosed at its optimal dilatation. This will prevent narrowing of the anastomoses. It is our belief that venous anastomoses are more likely to fail if this is not employed.

The anastomosis is completed in the same manner as the artery. Ensure bite sizes are 1.5× the thickness of the vessel wall and sutures are placed two needle thicknesses apart to allow maximum dilatation on clamp removal.

- The proximal clamp is opened first and the vessel slid gently out of the clamp. Blood should immediately fill the vessel back to the distal clip, having crossed the suture line.

- Open the distal clip and slide out the vein.

- Under low magnification, apply gentle pressure over the suture line with microsurgical swabs and wait for all bleeding to stop (**Figure 7.21**).

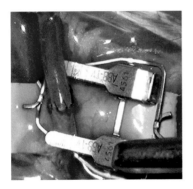 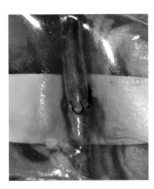

Figure 7.21 Venous clamp removal.

Copious bleeding must be considered a surgical failure, and another suture should be placed after reclamping and irrigating.

Assessment of venous patency

It is difficult to check that the vein is patent by simple observation. As described earlier, the 'milking' test is a very reliable tool.

The vein is occluded just proximal to the anastomosis with a pair of forceps, and the vessel is 'milked' for 3–4 mm proximally with another pair of forceps, which are then used to occlude the vessel.

This produces an empty length of vessel lying between the two occluding forceps.

If the anastomosis is patent, the vessel should rapidly refill as soon as the distal pair of forceps are released.

8 End-to-side anastomosis

Arterial preparation

In the rat and the chicken, the most convenient and simplest model for end-to-side anastomosis is to attach the end of the artery to the side of the vein.

Both vessels are prepared as per the dissection in Chapter 7. Slip the backing material under *both* vessels and instil a few drops of 2% procaine around the artery to prevent spasm (rat only).

● In the rat, using a single Acland clamp, occlude the artery as near to the inguinal ligament as possible, ligate the distal end of the artery at the junction with the superficial epigastric origin and transect the vessel straight across close to the tie (**Figure 8.1**).

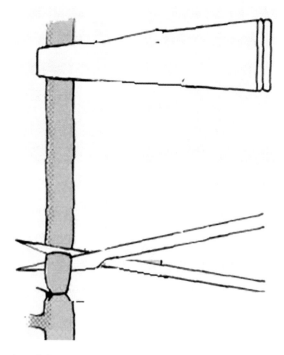

Figure 8.1 Transection of the artery.

● Remove adventitial tissue by the sleeve technique – see Chapter 7. The chicken artery can be transected at one end, It does not have a 'sleeve' of adventitia, so just trim any obvious adventitial tags.

DOI: 10.1201/9781003413080-8

- The approximating clamp is then positioned under the femoral vein as close to the inguinal ligament as practicable; it is important to clamp the vein here so that the anastomosis can be performed proximal to the point where the femoral artery has been divided so that no tension will be placed on the anastomotic site.

- With each clamp placed as far apart as possible, slide the vein into the proximal clip first and the distal clip next, as this ensures a ballooned vein.

This prevents possible damage to the opposite wall when a venotomy is created.

Performing the venotomy in the rat model

- Slide the clamps of the approximating clamp towards each other to release any tension. Bring the end of the prepared artery alongside the vein so that the artery lies in a gentle curve without tension.

The venotomy is created on the anterior venous wall and is size-matched to the outside diameter of the artery (**Figure 8.4**).

- This is achieved under top magnification by tenting the vein wall and creating the *smallest possible transverse* venotomy using Vannas scissors.

- Insert the closed tips of a No. D-5a forceps into the venotomy and, opening them slowly, longitudinally stretch the venotomy to the required size (the outside diameter of the artery) (**Figure 8.2**).

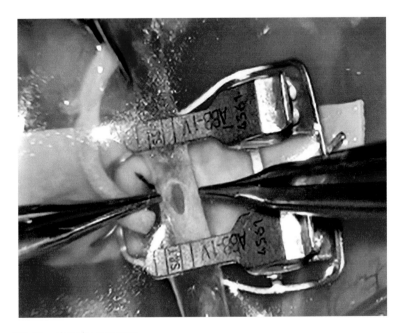

Figure 8.2 Completed venotomy.

Do not cut out a window of tissue in the rat vein to create a venotomy, as this invariably results in a larger venotomy than required.

A longitudinal venotomy tends to split the layers of the vessel wall and creates a rugged incision. The transverse cut produces a clean-edged venotomy, which immediately becomes elliptical due to the tension from the clamps. The venotomy is flushed out with heparinised saline.

This method of performing a venotomy does not work on the chicken model, as the vein is not as friable as the rat femoral vein, so the venotomy is extended using scissors.

General considerations

When performing a venotomy or arteriotomy, take into account vessel size. If the recipient vessel is smaller than the donor vessel, then it is important not to remove any tissue, as recipient flow will be compromised.

Always make the venotomy/arteriotomy length to the 'stretched' outside diameter of the donor vessel. This avoids narrowing at the anastomosis (see Chapter 6 for factors affecting anastomotic success).

Venous end-to-side anastomoses rely on perfectly matched venotomies to stay patent.

For arteriotomies, it is better to use a diamond knife or beaver blade to produce a straight non-jagged incision; however, these are not always on hand and scissors can be employed. A Potts-type microsurgical scissor with a 45°-angled blade can be used to extend arteriotomies and venotomies, leaving a clean incision.

Performing venotomies

This method works with the chicken model.

With veins, it is of the upmost importance to make the venotomy length match the *stretched* outside diameter of the donor vein. This avoids narrowing at the anastomosis.

Venous end-to-side anastomoses rely on perfectly matched venotomies to stay patent.

● To ensure a perfectly sized venotomy, make a transverse incision about half the size you will need.

● Place the first proximal stay suture in place and tie (**Figure 8.3**).

- Take the donor vein, gently stretch the lumen horizontally as far as it will easily go without damage and it is at this point that the venotomy will need extending to.

- The next stitch can be put in at this point to perfectly align the two vessel ends (**Figure 8.4**).

This method can also be used for arteriotomies.

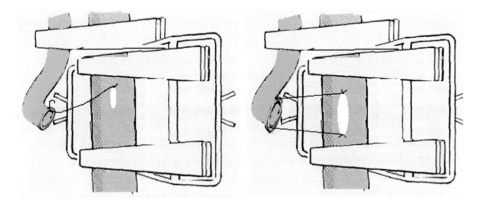

Figure 8.3 Placement of proximal stitch.   Figure 8.4 Extension of venotomy.

Performing arteriotomies

If you are confident about vessel matching, start the arteriotomy from the central point between the clamps. It can then be extended in either direction.

- With an end-to-side anastomosis of artery-to-artery, remove the adventitia minimally over the selected area. The vessel wall can be tented with No. D-5a forceps and either cut straight across with scissors or incised with the diamond or beaver knife.

If there are any tissue tags present, the resulting slight unevenness of the vessel edges will then be in the central part of the anastomosis and easily incorporated into the stitched area. If these are prominent, it may be necessary to remove a small diamond-shaped piece of vessel wall if scissors have been used to create the arteriotomy. The resulting tissue tags can then be removed, creating neat edges.

If the tissue tags occur at either end, it makes suturing them in much harder and stitch gaps can occur.

- The arteriotomy can then be incised in each direction with straight or Potts scissors.

Anterior wall of end-to-side artery to vein

● Arrange the end of the artery to lie alongside the venotomy ready for suturing. For each suture, take normal-sized bites out of both artery and vein, avoiding larger bites on the venous side, which can cause constriction.

● Space the sutures as close together as you would in an artery-to-artery anastomosis (one needle thickness apart).

● Place the first suture at the proximal end of the venotomy, passing the needle from the outside of the vein to the inside and thence from inside the artery to the outside. Pull the suture through until the edges of the vessels just meet and make a surgeon's knot, but leave one end long enough to attach to the farthest cleat of the clamp, but *do not* attach it at this stage (**Figure 8.5**).

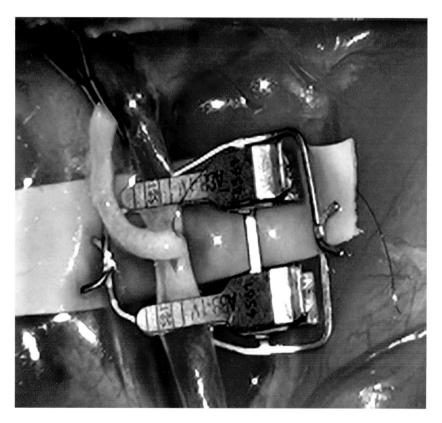

Figure 8.5 First stitch placement.

● Place the second suture at the opposite end of the venotomy, this time passing the needle outside of the artery to inside and thence inside the vein to outside. Again carefully tighten the suture, cutting both ends short.

● Place the third suture in the centre of the anterior wall (**Figure 8.6**).

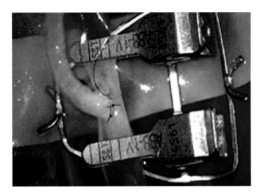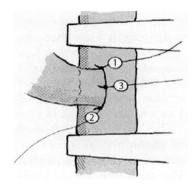

Figure 8.6 Anterior wall suture placement.

● Two additional sutures are placed in the front wall, one in each segment between the stay and holding sutures (**Figure 8.7**).

Remember to check each intermediate stitch *before* tying by examining the posterior wall, as it is very easy to catch the stitch through both walls.

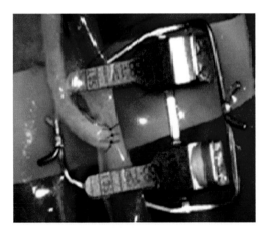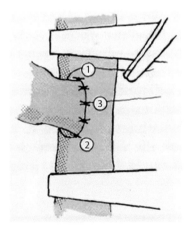

Figure 8.7 Completion of anterior wall.

Posterior wall

● To expose the posterior side, the long end of the first stay suture is passed under and around the back of the artery. This is used to retract the artery and expose the posterior wall for anastomosis and is attached to the cleat farthest from the anastomosis (**Figure 8.8**).

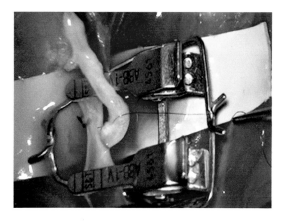
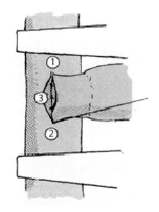

Figure 8.8 Placement of posterior stay suture.

Take care not to apply too much tension, as this can force the arterial and venous wall to lie too close to one another. This stitch is just used to hold the loop of artery gently out of the way.

The back wall can be completed in identical fashion to the front (**Figure 8.9**).

● Trim all long ends of knots and cut the stay sutures. Check that there are no obvious gaps when inspected at high magnification, and place extra sutures if the gaps look too large.

● After each stitch placement, gently raise the suture ends before tying to check that the anterior wall has not caught. Additionally keep the vein filled with saline, and this too will prevent anterior wall adherence.

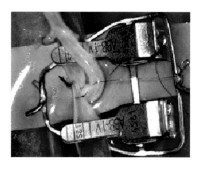
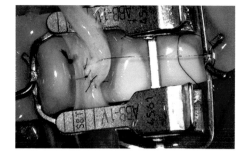

Figure 8.9 Completion of posterior wall.

Clamp removal

● Remove the approximating clamp from the vein, proximal clip first, followed by the distal clip (**Figure 8.10**).

● Inspect the posterior wall of the vein to ensure that no stitches have caught through.

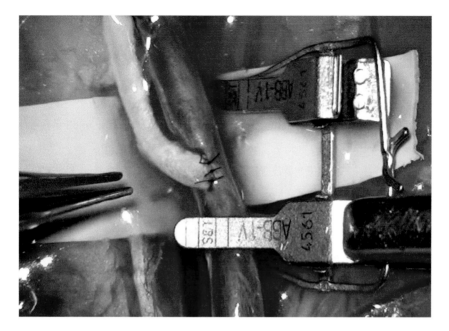

Figure 8.10 Proximal clamp removal.

Remove the single arterial clamp and check patency with the milk test.

If the anastomosis is patent, bright red blood should be observed mixing turbulently with venous blood in the vein.

- If the anastomosis is oozing, put gentle pressure over it with a damp swab for a few minutes before re-examining it under magnification.

- Finally instil a few drops of 2% procaine around the vessels to prevent or reverse any constriction.

Femoral artery to carotid loop (rat)

In this exercise the femoral artery in the rat is dissected free and anastomosed end to side into the carotid artery.

This will test dissection skills in the delicate neck area and the execution of two artery-to-artery end-to-side anastomoses.

The same exercise can be carried out in the chicken by harvesting a small tributary artery and anastomosing it to the chicken femoral artery.

The rat femoral triangle is exposed (Chapter 7) and the femoral artery dissected free.

- Place ties proximally and distally on the artery, taking as much length as possible. Transect at both ends, flush through and place into a pot of saline.

Carotid artery preparation

- Extend the rat's neck with an elastic band around the upper incisors and pin to the board. This extends the neck and makes the dissection easier.

- Make a midline incision 0.5 cm from below the mandible to 0.5 cm from the first rib.

- Blunt-dissect the fat free from below the incision and cut up the midline to expose the jugular vein.

- Retract the incision on the jugular side only.

- Tease apart the sternohyoid muscle and remove it to expose the carotid artery (**Figure 8.11**).

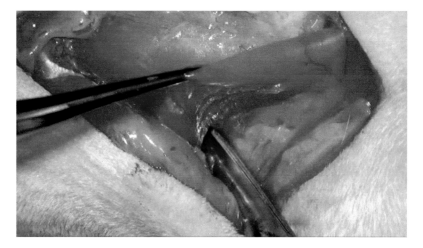

Figure 8.11 Exposure and removal of sternohyoid.

Take great care not to damage the vagus nerve.

- Free ~1 cm of carotid artery and place a plastic sheet behind the artery (**Figure 8.12**).

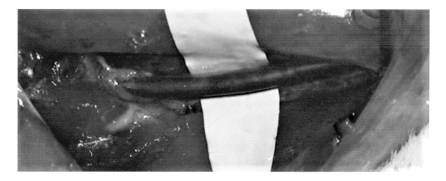

Figure 8.12 Rat carotid artery dissection.

Take great care when handling the carotid artery, as the vessel wall is thinner and under more pressure than the femoral artery.

- Clamp the carotid artery as proximally and distally as possible using single clamps.
- Trim off excess adventitia.
- Towards the distal clamp make the first arteriotomy using Vannas scissors and flush with heparinised saline.
- Enlarge the arteriotomy as necessary to equal the diameter of the femoral artery (**Figure 8.13**).

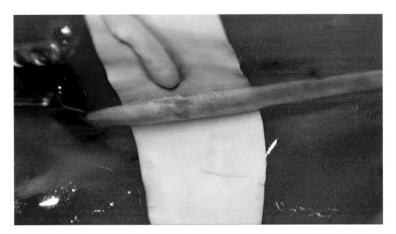

Figure 8.13 Enlarged arteriotomy.

Anastomose the anterior wall using interrupted 10/0 nylon stitches (8/0 for chicken).

- Place the stay sutures at 180° into the femoral and carotid arteries.
- Take a backhand stitch for the second stay suture (**Figure 8.14**).

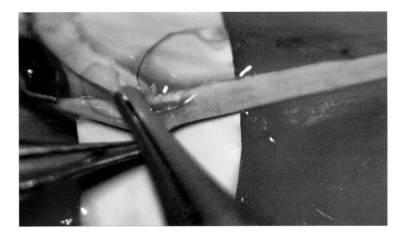

Figure 8.14 Second stay suture.

- Complete the anterior wall with three further stitches; if you are not confident, check each stitch before tying.

- Flip the femoral artery over to expose the posterior wall; complete with three further stitches.

- Make sure there is a good 'curve' to the femoral artery, ensuring there is no tension or twisting of the vessel.

- Perform the second arteriotomy in the same manner as the first (**Figure 8.15**).

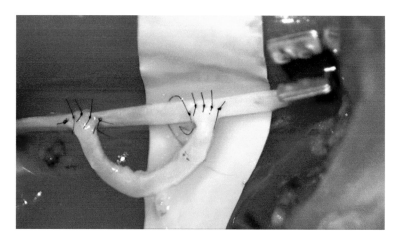

Figure 8.15 Second anastomosis.

- Tie off the carotid artery with 7/0 silk midway between the anastomoses.

- Remove the distal clamp and wait for the anastomoses to stop oozing and then remove the proximal clamp; test flow in the distal carotid and femoral artery with the 'milk' test (**Figure 8.16**).

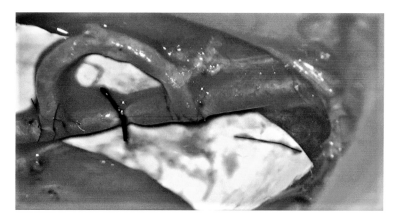

Figure 8.16 Completed carotid loop.

9 Interpositional vein graft

Much of clinical microvascular surgery involves repair of avulsed and damaged vessels which have to be resected. It is preferable to interpose a vein graft with two anastomoses rather than risk a single anastomosis being subjected to longitudinal tension.

A segment of vein can be used to bridge a gap between the divided ends of either an artery or another vein. The suturing technique is essentially the same as that described for the end-to-end anastomosis (**Figure 9.1**).

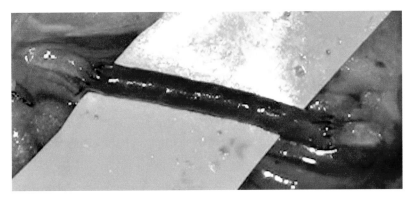

Figure 9.1 Epigastric vein graft in the rat.

The only real difficulty likely to be encountered is discrepancy in size, which complicates the suturing itself and may lead to constriction or, conversely, ballooning with consequent rheological complications and added risk of thrombosis (**Figure 9.2**).

See Chapter 6 for factors affecting anastomotic success.

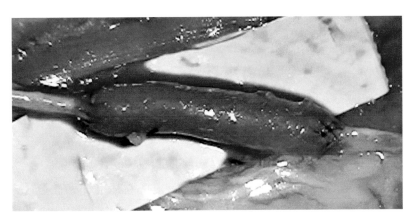

Figure 9.2 Femoral (discrepant size) vein graft in the rat.

DOI: 10.1201/9781003413080-9

This chapter will describe vein grafts that match the recipient vessel size and those that involve discrepancy.

In each of these methods great care must be taken not to suture the front wall of the vessel to the back. It is also very important to ensure that the vessels are under no tension, or the smaller vessel is likely to tear.

For the discrepant vein exercise, the ends of the vessel are cut straight so the maximum size difference is obtained. This will enhance the difficulty and make suture placement paramount (see Chapter 6 for alternative matching techniques). Clinical situations will dictate which method is utilised.

Vessel preparation for a discrepant-sized vein graft

In the rat model, a segment of the femoral vein is removed, reversed (so that the valves open in the direction of the blood flow) and sutured end-to-end between the divided ends of the femoral artery. When fully dilated, this vein is approximately twice the diameter of the femoral artery.

In the chicken you will not need to place single clamps on the artery, as the vessel is non-viable.

For clinical work, it is important that valves open in the direction of blood flow. The tied-off profunda femoris vein on the rat femoral vein acts as a marker for orientation.

- Ligate the vein with a 7/0 tie at each end and divide close to the proximal tie (**Figure 9.3**).

- Flush the vein but leave the distal end attached until the artery is prepared (it is very easy to lose the vein once detached!).

- Clamp the artery at each end and divide the artery in the centre.

- Flush out and remove the adventitia. The natural retraction of the arterial segments creates space, so it is unnecessary to excise any artery (**Figure 9.4**).

The first anastomosis is slightly more difficult, as the double clamp is not stable and can move around. Take time to place the clamp in such a way as to minimise this. In the rat ensure the operative field is open enough to place four clamps in a row.

- Place the proximal artery into the top of the double clamp (**Figure 9.5**).

- Detach the vein close to the distal tie, reverse it, then place it onto the background material and flush. This prevents any twisting of the vessel.

- Irrigate well and 'float' the vein into the clamp. This will prevent kinks and twisting when clamping (**Figure 9.6**).

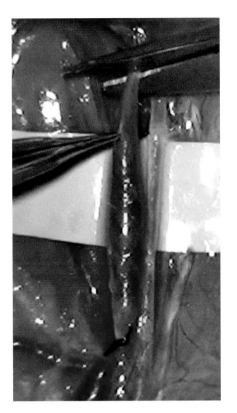

Figure 9.3 Vein preparation.

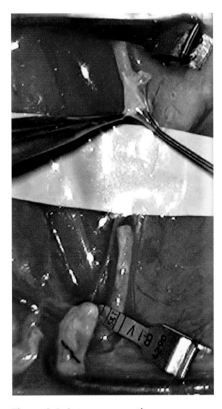

Figure 9.4 Artery preparation.

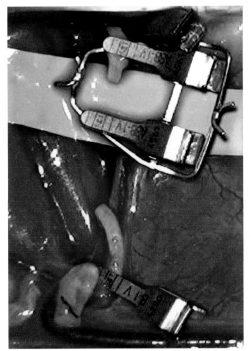

Figure 9.5 Artery clamping.

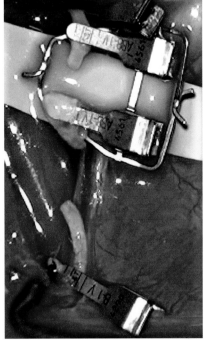

Figure 9.6 Vein clamping.

Tips for success

Place sutures at the same relative position (the 120° point on the artery must be aligned with the 120° point on the vein) around the circumference of both vessels, or gaps will be left on insertion of the final sutures due to misalignment.

To compensate for the difference in the thickness of the vessel walls, the artery has a normal bite size (1.5× the thickness of its walls), but the vein also has an 'arterial' bite size (this slightly bunches the vein wall to make it thicker and ensures it seals against the arterial edge) **(Figure 9.7)**.

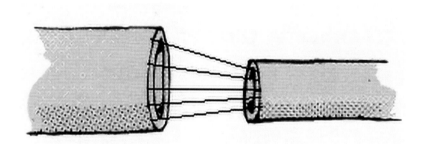

Figure 9.7 120° to 120° suture placement.

- Following placement of the first two stay sutures, release the distal clamp and pull the vein slightly taut and then reclamp **(Figure 9.8)**.

This opens up the anastomotic site and makes suture placement more obvious.

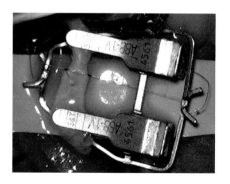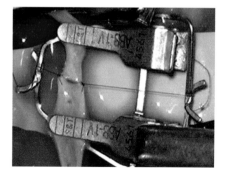

Figure 9.8 Slight tension is applied to open the anastomotic site.

- Keep the vein filled with saline to facilitate suture placement and to prevent catching the opposite vessel wall.

- Complete the end-to-end anastomosis with sutures spaced as if for an arterial anastomosis (one needle width apart) to prevent leakage (**Figure 9.9**).

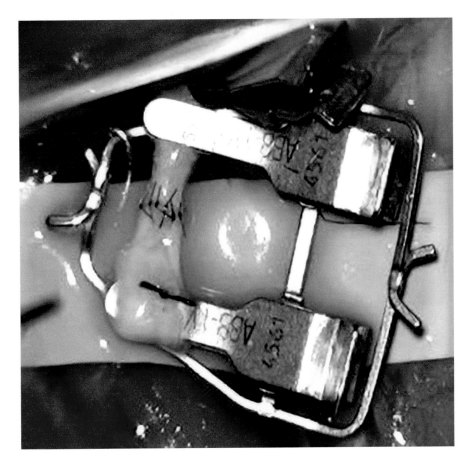

Figure 9.9 Completion of first anastomosis.

- Do not test the patency of this first anastomosis by releasing the proximal single clamp; thrombosis will occur by the time the second anastomosis has been completed.

Distal anastomosis preparation

- When the proximal anastomosis is complete, remove the approximating clamp and flush through with heparinised saline.
- Reposition the double clamp so that the distal end of the vein graft can be secured in the proximal clip.

- Secure the distal segment of the artery into the distal clip. Ensure the vein and artery are relaxed and not twisted or kinked (**Figure 9.10**).

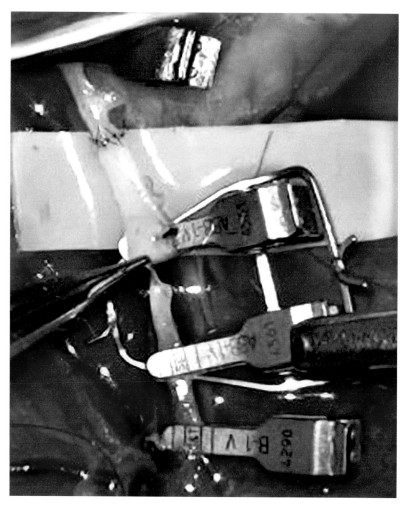

Figure 9.10 Arterial clamping.

- Complete the second (distal) anastomosis.
  - The distal vein may be wider than the proximal (the rat femoral vein is not a straight tube; it may be necessary to place more sutures in the posterior distal anastomosis).

Clamp removal

- Remove the double clamp.
- Remove the distal clamp.

● Apply pressure and wait for bleeding to cease.

● Remove the proximal clamp (**Figure 9.11**).

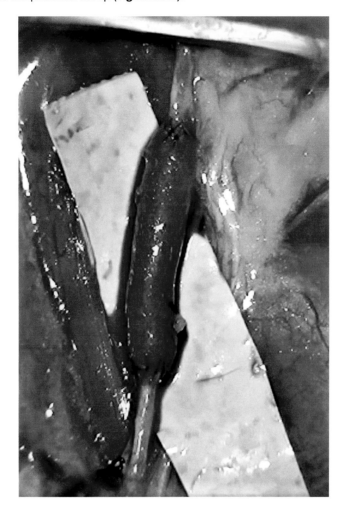

Figure 9.11 Clamp removal.

● *Patency*: A gentle ooze should soon stop. For a pulsatile leak, reapply single clamps to the distal and proximal artery. Flush through the gap to remove all blood. Fix the gap with a stitch and then remove the clamps.

● *Warning*: Placing a stitch into a pulsatile leak will lead to a misplaced stitch and more importantly thrombus will be 'locked in' if the static blood is not removed and anastomotic failure will ensue. Do *not* milk the vein, as it is easily damaged and under arterial pressure.

To test patency, milk test the proximal artery and compare it to the distal arterial flow.

Epigastric vein graft in the rat

In the rat model, a segment of superficial epigastric vein is removed, reversed and sutured end-to-end between the divided ends of the femoral artery. When fully dilated, this vein is approximately the same diameter as the femoral artery.

The test in this exercise is gentle handling and identifying the lumen of a very friable 1 mm vein.

● Expose the femoral triangle as before and prepare the femoral artery.

● Gently dissect free 1 cm of the epigastric vein, ensuring there is no tension on the vein.

● For clinical work, it is important that valves open in the direction of blood flow. Place a 10/0 marker stitch near one end to identify orientation before resection.

● Ligate the vein with a 7/0 tie at each end and divide close to the proximal tie (**Figure 9.12**).

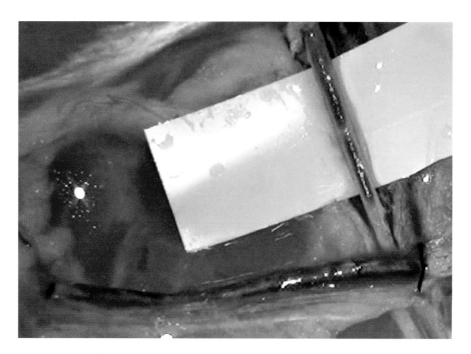

Figure 9.12 Vein dissection.

● Flush the vein but leave the distal end attached until the artery is prepared (it is very easy to lose the vein once detached) (**Figure 9.13**).

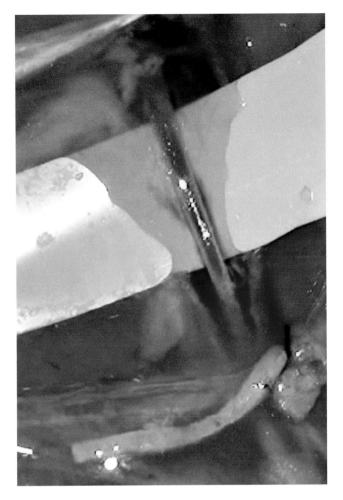

Figure 9.13 Vein preparation.

The method from now on is similar to that of the discrepant vein graft.

- The superficial epigastric vein is now divided at its distal end, and the graft is laid alongside the approximating clamp with the marker stitch identifying the orientation.

- Irrigate the vein with heparinised saline to eliminate kinks.

- Open the distal clip of the approximating clamp and slide in the vein graft with enough length protruding proximally to carry out the anastomosis comfortably (**Figure 9.14**).

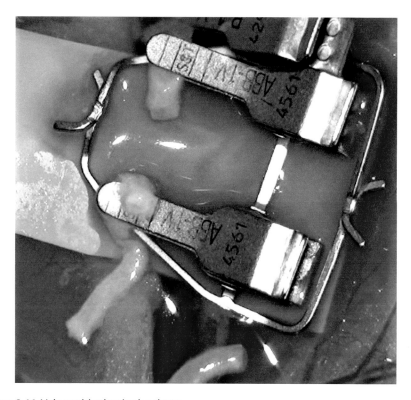

Figure 9.14 Vein positioning in the clamp.

- Complete an end-to-end anastomosis with sutures spaced as closely as if it were an arterial end-to-end anastomosis to prevent leakage after high-pressure blood flow is restored.

When suturing, take arterial-sized bites from the artery and vein-sized bites from the vein to prevent narrowing of the anastomosis.

- When the proximal anastomosis is complete, remove the approximating clamp and flush through with heparinised saline (**Figure 9.15**).

- Reposition the double clamp so that the distal end of the vein graft can be secured in the proximal clip and the distal segment of the artery can be held in the distal clip.

    - Do not test the patency of this first anastomosis by releasing the proximal single clamp, as thrombosis will occur by the time the distal anastomosis has been completed.

- The vein will expand to its full length on reflow, so before the distal anastomosis, shorten the vein length by a third to prevent kinking (**Figure 9.16**).

- Complete the distal anastomosis and remove the approximating clamp.

- Remove the distal clamp and allow time for blood to flow back across both anastomoses.

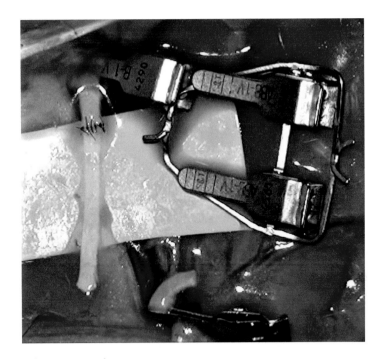

Figure 9.15 First anastomosis.

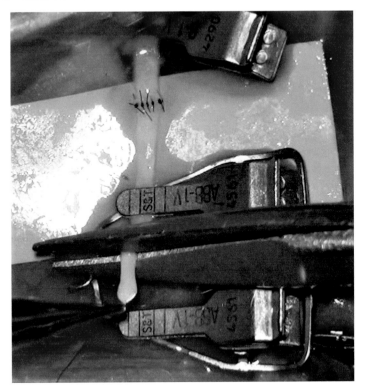

Figure 9.16 Shortening vein length.

- Once any leakage has ceased, remove the proximal single clamp.

- Apply gentle pressure for a minute before examining the two suture lines for leaks and testing patency (**Figure 9.17**).

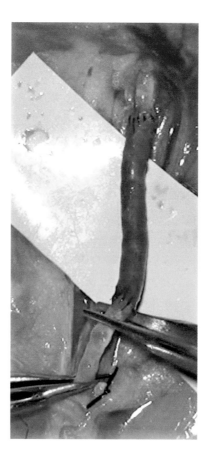

Figure 9.17 **Patency.**

- *Patency*: Test patency by 'milking' the distal artery – the flow should match the proximal artery. The vein is under pressure and friable, so do not attempt the milk test on it. A gentle ooze should soon stop.

- *Warning*: For a pulsatile leak, reapply single clamps to the distal and proximal artery. Flush through the gap to remove all blood. Fix the gap with a stitch and then remove the clamps. Placing a stitch into a pulsatile leak will lead to a misplaced stitch and more importantly thrombus will be 'locked in' if the static blood is not removed and anastomotic failure will ensue.

10 Vessels under 1 mm

Rat and chicken models

For these exercises on vessels below 1 mm in diameter, the models utilised are the chicken thigh and the groin flap in the rat.

- In the chicken, the smaller vessels can be found branching off the artery and vein at the proximal and distal ends and also about halfway along the length.

- In rats, a groin flap raised on the superficial epigastric vessels provides a suitable model in which to develop skills for clinical free-flap procedures (**Figure 10.1**).

The confidence gained in anastomosing and achieving patency in vessels of this size is not wasted when returning to the larger vessels normally encountered in clinical practice.

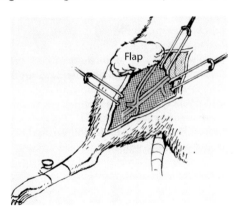

Figure 10.1 Rat groin flap.

Chicken model

For dissection practice, the chicken tributary vessels are dissected free, cut and anastomosed.

Rat groin flap

A rectangular area 4 cm × 2 cm is marked out on the depilated skin. An incision using a scalpel is made around the whole flap.

The flap is lifted with microtoothed forceps at the anterior medial corner and then raised, together with its vessel-bearing fat pad, by blunt dissection with round-tipped bow scissors.

DOI: 10.1201/9781003413080-10

Great care must be taken when cutting through the inguinal fat pad at the posterior border of the flap, as it usually contains vessel branches. These vessels can be contained within the flap if a larger ratio of fat to skin is taken in this area.

It is important that the whole of the flap is freed from any adherent tissue and that it is completely isolated on the superficial epigastric pedicle. If the flap remains attached by any peripheral vessels during the vascular anastomosis, it will become congested and fail.

However good your anastomotic skills are, the vessels will not flow if damaged during the preparation stage.

Once the flap has been freed of all connections except the vascular pedicle, it is elevated and placed skin side down onto a supportive bed of damp swabs, *ensuring that the pedicle is under no tension* (**Figure 10.2**).

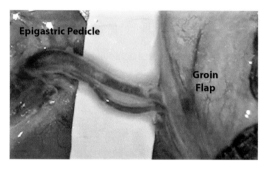

Figure 10.2 Dissected groin flap.

The flap is positioned so that it is at the same level as the rat leg to ensure that the anastomotic area is kept as flat as possible.

This achieves two objectives:

● The prevention of blood pooling within the flap, which can lead to thrombosis

● The maintenance of focus of the whole of the vessel bed when using high magnification

The flap is then covered with damp swabs, as is the donor site, to prevent desiccation.

Vessel dissection for end-to-end anastomosis of epigastric vessels

Epigastric artery and vein

● The superficial epigastric artery and vein are separated from each other for a distance of ~1 cm (from the junction with the femoral vessels to the bifurcation into the fat pad of the flap).

● Background material is then inserted underneath both vessels.

However carefully the dissection may have been executed, the artery will spasm, and once divided, the arterial lumen can be difficult to identify. (Chicken artery will not spasm, as the tissue is non-viable.)

● *Before* the microvascular clamps can be applied, the artery must be fully dilated. There are three methods that can be used:

Cut down to the femoral artery *distal* to the epigastric junction and occlude the femoral artery with a single Acland clamp. This diverts the flow into the epigastric artery.

Instil a few drops of 2% procaine onto the artery and then wait for a few minutes.

Gently massage along the length of the vessel using microforceps.

This is a very effective method, but *great care* must be taken not to crush the intima (**Figure 10.3**).

Take tension off the vessels to prevent further spasm.

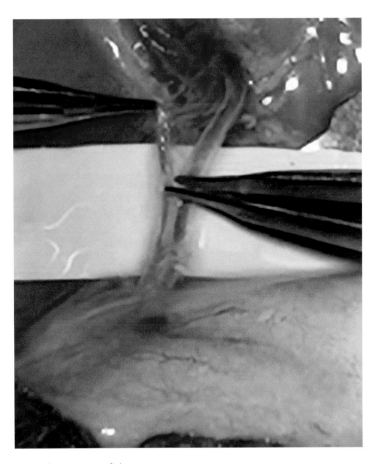

Figure 10.3 Gentle massage of the artery.

Once the artery is *fully* dilated and pulsating, the vessels can be clamped.

- A single Acland clamp is applied across *both* the artery and vein at the proximal end.
- The vessels are then divided at their midpoints.
- The proximal vein stump is flushed with heparinised saline and kept moist (**Figure 10.4**).

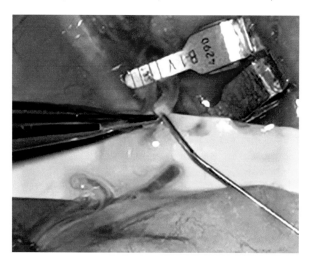

Figure 10.4 Vessel irrigation.

- The artery is gently 'stroked' with the Rycroft cannula to remove the blood and the adventitial sleeve removed.
- The lumen is dilated with one tip of the forceps (**Figure 10.5**).

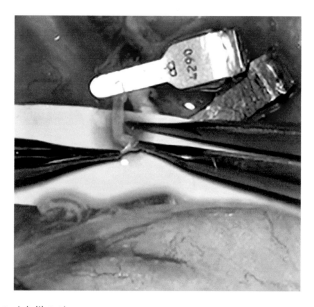

Figure 10.5 Arterial dilatation.

It is important to perfuse the flap with 1 mL of heparinised saline. Failure to do this will result in a thrombosed flap.

- The flap is perfused via the epigastric artery using a 30-g Rycroft cannula on a 1 mL syringe.

- Place the vessels onto a damp swab so that the lumens are facing the operator.

- Flush the end of the vein with heparinised saline. This ensures that the vein lumen does not adhere to itself and allow pressure to build up within the flap during perfusion (**Figure 10.6**).

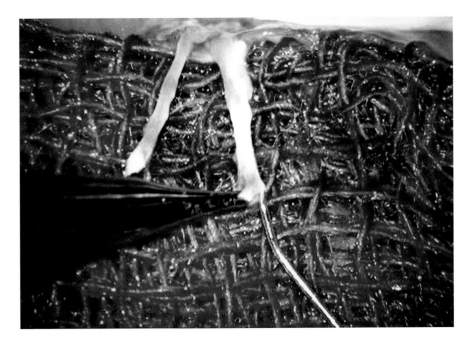

Figure 10.6 Vein flushing.

- Remove the arterial adventitia using the sleeve technique. Insert one tip of the forceps into the arterial lumen to dilate.

- Grasp the edge of the arterial adventitia. Allow a stream of heparinised saline to flow from the cannula at the moment of insertion. This will dilate and hold open the lumen (**Figure 10.7**).

- Grip the distal artery and cannula with the forceps and perfuse the flap with 1 mL of heparinised saline (the damaged part of the artery will be removed before the anastomosis).

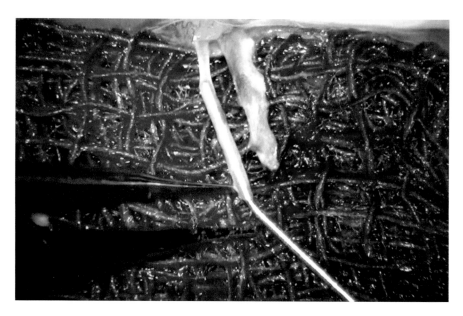

Figure 10.7 Arterial cannulation.

Epigastric arterial anastomosis

The artery is anastomosed end-to-end with 10/0 or 11/0 monofilament suture using the triangulation technique. Full magnification (at least 16–20×) should be used whilst passing the needle and at least 10× magnification when tying the knots.

- The double clamp is applied to the artery so that there is plenty of vessel length contained between the clamps to ensure adequate working space. The end of the artery is trimmed to remove any tissue that may have been damaged during the cannulation procedure.

The key to perfecting anastomoses in small vessels is the accurate placement of the first two stitches. Any misalignment will lead to failure.

- Each suture should be checked by the insertion of the forcep tip into the posterior wall *before* tying, as it can be very difficult to rectify mistakes in such small vessels once they are tied. The artery normally requires approximately seven stitches (**Figure 10.8**).

- Place two stay sutures: Two on the anterior wall and three on the posterior.

During the anastomosis, it is crucial to keep the vessel wet, as any desiccation leads to adherence of the vessel lumen, which provides a prime site for platelet aggregation. Be aware also of the vessels and tissues *outside* of the clamps becoming dry.

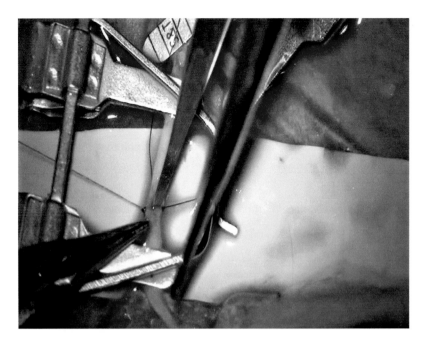

Figure 10.8 Stitch checking.

● On completion of the arterial anastomoses, the approximating clamp is removed and the area irrigated (**Figure 10.9**).

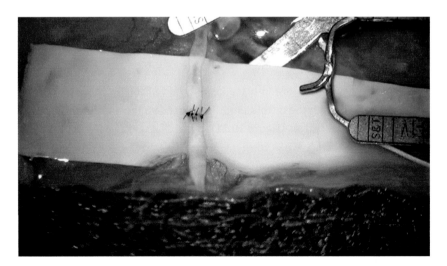

Figure 10.9 Double clamp removal.

Do *not* attempt to test patency in the artery at this stage, as static blood present within the arterial anastomosis and the flap will lead to thrombosis during the time taken to complete the venous anastomosis.

Epigastric venous anastomosis

Use 10/0 or 11/0 nylon suture.

- To complete the venous anastomosis, a second piece of background material is placed over the artery and underneath the vein. This helps to prevent desiccation and physical damage to the artery from the clamp.

- The approximating clamp is applied to the vein, ensuring that there is no tension on the flap and that there is sufficient vessel length between the individual clamps of the approximator.

It is crucial to accurately place the first two stay sutures to avoid misalignment.

- Place as much horizontal tension as you can so that the vein is anastomosed as if fully dilated (**Figure 10.10**).

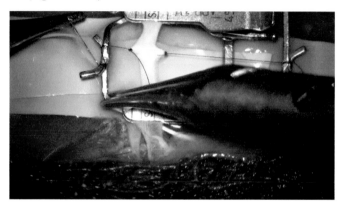

Figure 10.10 Horizontal tension.

- Once the first two sutures are in place, adjust the tension on the anastomosis by pulling the vein through the distal clamp. This opens up the anastomosis and helps to visualise the vessel edges (**Figure 10.11**).

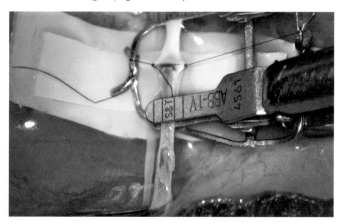

Figure 10.11 Adjusting tension.

- Check each stitch before tying to ensure the back wall is not caught.

- Make sure each stitch is placed two needle widths apart.

- Place two stay sutures: Two on the anterior wall and three on the posterior.

Trust the method! Too many sutures leads to a 'waist' at the anastomosis and therefore compromised flow.

- On completion, the approximating clamp is removed and the area irrigated.

- The top piece of background material is removed and any tension on the flap and vessels reduced.

- The single clamp occluding both vessels is removed and a few drops of 2% procaine are administered to the artery to alleviate any potential spasm.

- Patency can be confirmed by the milk test on the vein (**Figure 10.12**). Testing the artery will cause damage, so leave it alone.

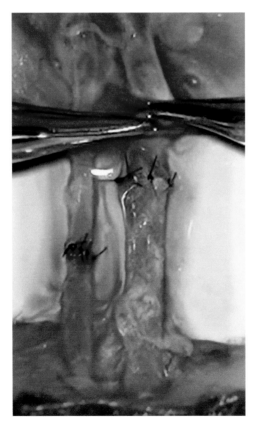

Figure 10.12 Patency test.

Ensure all tension is taken off both vessels. The artery cannot pulsate under tension and may lead to flap failure.

Vessel dissection for end-to-side anastomosis of epigastric vessels

The groin flap is dissected free as before, but the epigastric vessels are divided at their junction with the femoral vessels to give a longer pedicle. The flap is then flushed as before.

Femoral artery preparation

The flap is laid adjacent to the femoral vessels, ensuring there is no tension on the epigastric vessels.

- Single Acland clamps are applied to the proximal and distal femoral artery (**Figure 10.13**).
- The double clamp is applied to the femoral artery.
- The epigastric artery is shortened to remove the damaged tip caused by the flap irrigation.
- The femoral artery adventitial window is removed.
- The arteriotomy is performed with Vannas scissors.

Gentle vessel handling is paramount. Injury at this stage will lead to failed anastomoses.

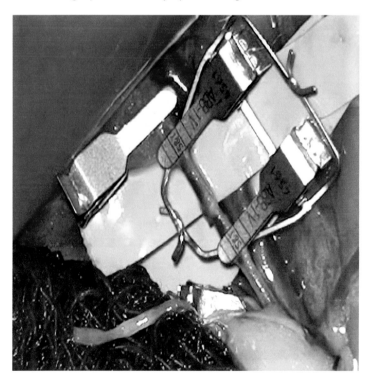

Figure 10.13 Femoral clamping.

Femoral artery anastomosis

During the anastomosis, it is crucial to keep the vessel wet, as any desiccation leads to adherence of the vessel lumen, which provides a prime site for platelet aggregation. Be aware also of the vessels and tissues *outside* of the clamps becoming dry.

● Perform the femoral arteriotomy and dilate the epigastric artery.

● Place two stay sutures (10/0 or 11/0 nylon), leaving the end of the proximal suture long enough to reach the farthest clamp cleats.

● Complete the anterior anastomosis with three sutures. Pass the long suture under the epigastric artery (**Figure 10.14**).

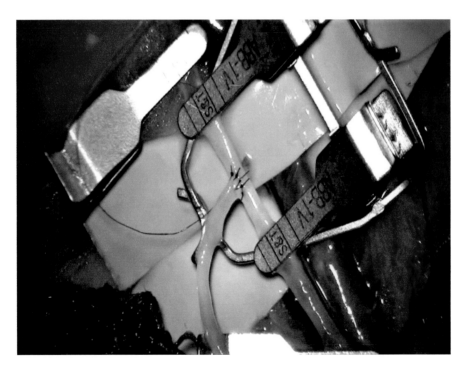

Figure 10.14 Anterior wall.

● Attach the long stay suture to the farthest cleat to stabilise the vessel for the posterior wall (**Figure 10.15**).

● Complete the posterior wall with three sutures (**Figure 10.16**).

● On completion of the arterial anastomoses, the approximating clamp is removed and the area irrigated.

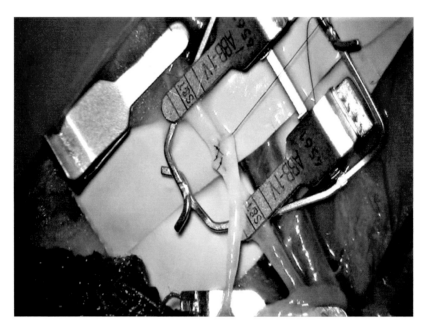

Figure 10.15 Attachment of stay suture.

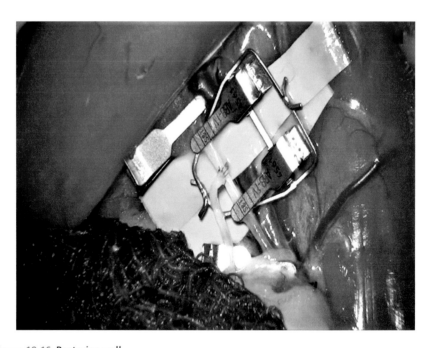

Figure 10.16 Posterior wall.

Do *not* attempt to test patency in the artery at this stage, as static blood present within the arterial anastomosis and the flap will lead to thrombosis during the time taken to complete the venous anastomosis.

Femoral vein anastomosis

The surface of the vein is cleaned of any connective tissue to give a smooth surface, but do not overstrip.

- The double Acland clamp is applied to the femoral vein.

- The epigastric vein is aligned to the femoral vein.

- The venotomy is performed transversely with Vannas scissors.

- The vein is stretched horizontally as far as it will go and the venotomy enlarged accordingly.

The key to a successful venous anastomosis is ensuring that the vein is anastomosed whilst at its most stretched (dilated) state.

During the anastomosis, it is crucial to keep the vessel wet, as any desiccation leads to adherence of the vessel lumen, which provides a prime site for platelet aggregation. Be aware also of the vessels and tissues *outside* of the clamps becoming dry.

- Place two stay sutures (10/0 or 11/0 nylon), leaving the end of the proximal suture long enough to reach the farthest clamp cleats.

- Complete the anterior anastomosis with three sutures. Pass the long suture under the epigastric vein (**Figure 10.17**).

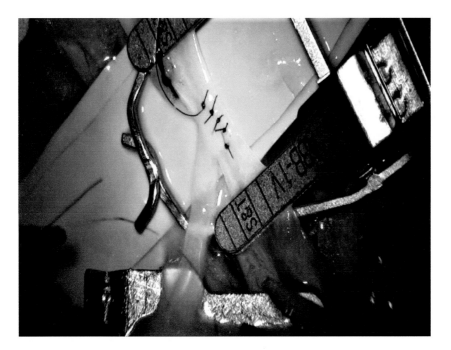

Figure 10.17 Anterior wall.

● Attach the long stay suture to the farthest cleat to stabilise the vessel for the posterior wall.

● Complete the posterior wall with three sutures (**Figure 10.18**).

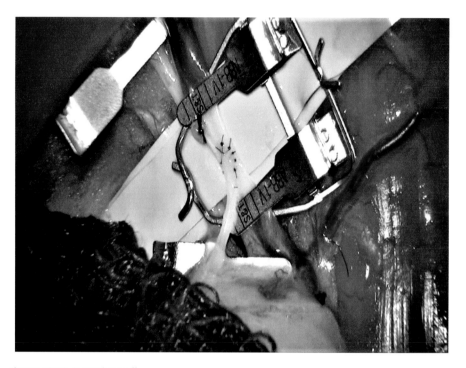

Figure 10.18 Posterior wall.

● On completion of the venous anastomoses, the approximating clamp is removed and the area irrigated.

● Remove the venous double clamp.

● Remove the distal arterial single clamp.

● Remove the proximal arterial single clamp.

● Apply a damp swab until oozing stops (**Figure 10.19**).

● Check patency with the milk test (**Figure 10.20**).

Do *not* be tempted to use the milk test on the epigastric artery. The vessel is very delicate and could be damaged. Patency is assessed by venous outflow.

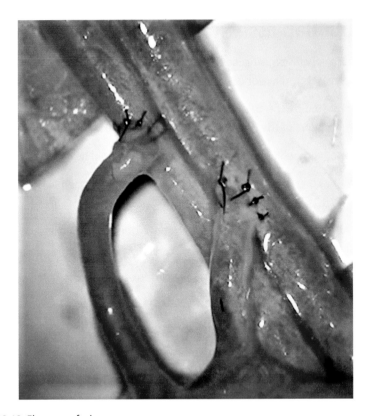

Figure 10.19 Flap reperfusion.

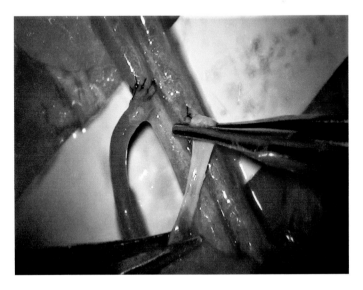

Figure 10.20 Patency test.

Rat groin flap assessment

The vessels are very unforgiving, so the aim is to get it right first time. A salvage operation of these vessels rarely works.

Success is indicated by the colour of the flap. It should turn pink with oozing of the vessels at the borders of the flap and feel warm to the touch.

- If the flap remains white, the patency of the artery should be checked.

- If it becomes congested, cyanosed and cool to the touch, then venous patency is suspect.

- If the vessels are not patent, it is best to remove both anastomoses, resect back to healthy tissue and repeat the exercise.

- If there is a Doppler available, this can be used to assess patency.

If the flap appears healthy, it is advisable to return the flap to its original position, ensuring that the pedicle is not stressed or kinked and to cover it with a damp swab. The flap should be left for about 20 minutes, as any problems likely to arise usually manifest themselves within this time.

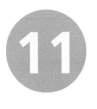

11 Anastomosis with single clamps

These exercises can be performed on both the chicken and the rat. Vessels are exposed as before.

Anastomosis with single clamps

One side up

The idea here is to place the first stitch in the centre of the posterior wall and gradually work around to the anterior wall. This method works best for thicker-walled vessels, where the lumen is more likely to stay open (**Figure 11.1**).

With this method, suture alignment and placement can be more difficult, particularly for veins, as they can be friable and tend to 'collapse' when transected.

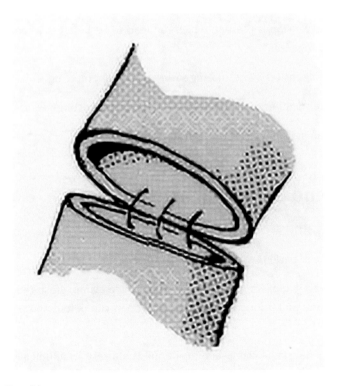

Figure 11.1 One side up.

DOI: 10.1201/9781003413080-11

Double versus single clamps

Given the option, it is better to use an Acland double-approximating clamp. However, not every establishment has these, so learning to use two single clamps instead is valuable.

We recommend students be familiar with the double clamp application before attempting the procedure with the single.

Double clamp advantages

● Takes longitudinal tension off the vessel.

● Allows the vessel to have adequate tension throughout the anastomosis, ensuring accurate suture placement.

● Allows easy access to the posterior wall when checking suture placement.

● Negates the need for an assistant to hold the sutures when required.

Single clamp disadvantages

● Longitudinal tension is present, which can lead to tissue tears when bringing the vessel ends together.

● All horizontal tension is lost, making suture placement more difficult.

● Suture placement has to be accurate, as checking the posterior wall is difficult.

● May need an assistant to provide tension.

End-to-end arterial anastomosis

Applying clamps

● Slide a piece of backing material under the artery.

● With the clamp appliers, apply the proximal single clamp, grasp the artery by its adventitia and pull it longitudinally into the open clip before allowing it to close (**Figure 11.2**).

● Open the distal single clamp and again pull the artery longitudinally toward the proximal clamp, slide it into the clamp and allow this to close.

Place the single clamps as far apart as you can.

This manoeuvre ensures a relaxed length of artery between each clip. Do not twist the vessel, and ensure that it is held at the *tip* of the clamp; clamping the vessel nearer the clamp hinge may lead to vessel slippage.

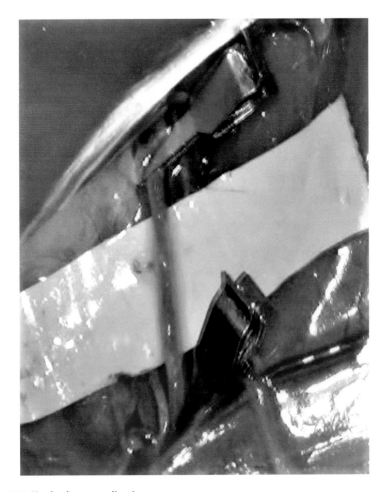

Figure 11.2 Single clamp application.

This method uses the 120° or triangulation technique (described in Chapter 7).

● Transect, flush and remove the adventitia.

● Place the first 120° stitch with a double throw and *gently* bring the edges together, ensuring there are no tears in the wall (**Figure 11.3**).

● Complete the stitch with two single throws and leave the proximal end of the stitch long.

● Place the second 120° stitch in the same way as the first, leaving the proximal end long (**Figure 11.4**).

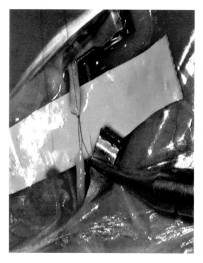

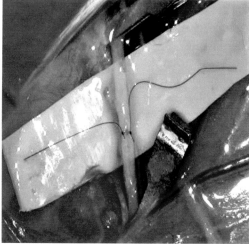

Figure 11.3 First stitch placement. Figure 11.4 Stay sutures.

● Apply single clamps to the long ends. These act as 'weights' to help add horizontal tension (an assistant can replace the single clamp 'weights' if a suitably trained individual is available).

● Place the third stitch with two single throws in the middle of the anterior wall, leaving the proximal end of the suture long (**Figure 11.5**).

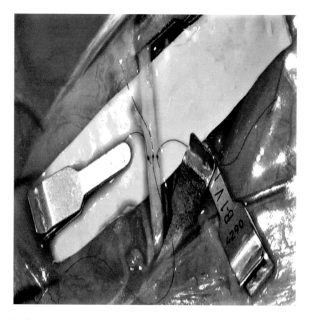

Figure 11.5 Single clamp 'weights'.

- On the anterior wall, place another stitch on either side of the central stitch, using the central stitch to give some tension.

- Remove the single clamp weights. Pass one stay suture under and one over to reveal the posterior wall. Replace the single clamp weights.

- Place a central stitch into the posterior wall, leaving the proximal end long. Remove the right single clamp weight onto the central stitch to give tension **(Figure 11.6)**.

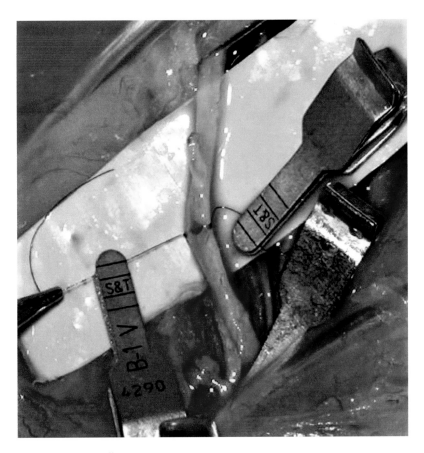

Figure 11.6 Posterior wall exposure.

- Move the single clamp over to the left and place two further sutures into the right hand gap.

- Move the single clamp over to the right and place the last two stitches into the left hand gap **(Figure 11.7)**.

- Remove the distal clamp, wait for oozing to stop and then remove the proximal clamp **(Figure 11.8)**.

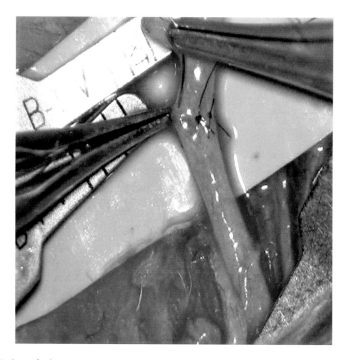

Figure 11.7 Completing anastomosis.

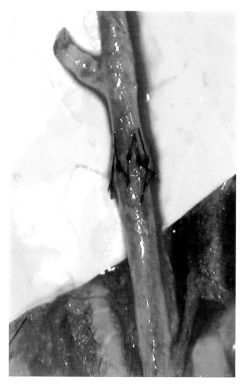

Figure 11.8 Completed anastomosis.

End-to-end venous anastomosis

This uses the same 120° or triangulation technique as for the artery.

- Apply single clamps to the vein distal end first.

- Place as proximally and distally as possible.

- Transect, flush and remove any obvious connective tissue.

- Place the first 120° stitch with a double throw and gently bring the edges together, ensuring there are no tears in the wall.

- Complete the stitch with two single throws and leave the proximal end of the stitch long.

- Place the second 120° stitch in the same way as the first, leaving the proximal end long.

- Apply single clamps to the long ends – these act as 'weights' to help add horizontal tension.

- Place a third stitch with two single throws in the middle of the anterior wall, leaving the proximal end of the suture long.

- On the anterior wall, place another stitch on either side of the central stitch, using the central stitch to give some tension (**Figure 11.9**).

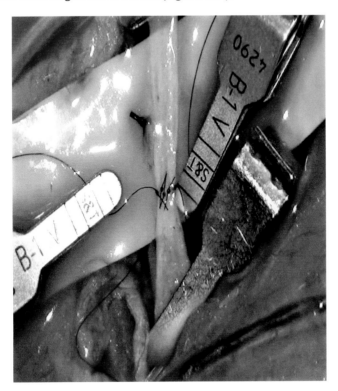

Figure 11.9 Anterior wall anastomosis.

- Remove the single clamp weights. Pass one stay suture under and one over to reveal the posterior wall.

- Replace the single clamp weights onto the long ends and place a central stitch, leaving the proximal end long.

- Remove the right single clamp weight onto the central stitch to give tension.

- Place another central stitch into the vein portion, leaving the proximal end long, and add another stitch on either side.

- Move the weight clamp over to the left and place another central stitch to the vein portion, leaving the proximal end long, and add another stitch on either side (**Figure 11.10**).

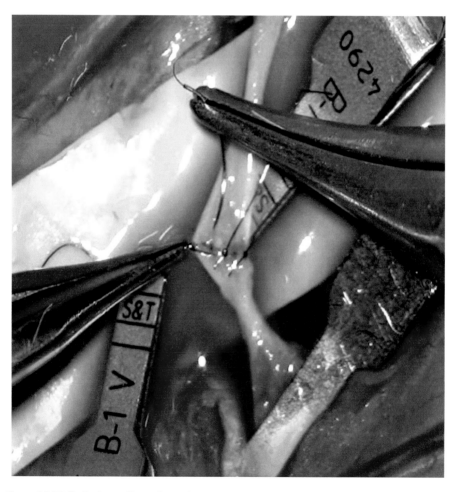

Figure 11.10 Posterior wall anastomosis.

- Irrigate vein, remove the proximal clamp, wait for oozing to stop and then remove the distal clamp (**Figure 11.11**).

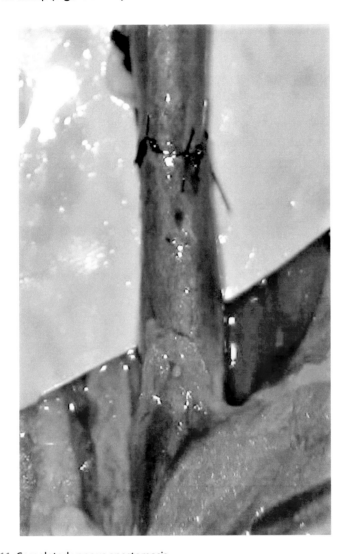

Figure 11.11 Completed venous anastomosis.

When using the double clamp, only five stitches are placed into the venous posterior wall; because of difficulties in alignment with the single clamp method, more may be needed. Take care to take very small stitch bites (1.5× the thickness of the vessel wall) to avoid narrowing at the anastomosis.

12 Continuous suturing techniques

In this module, the femoral artery and vein in the rat are dissected and anastomosed with a continuous suturing technique. The same exercises can be carried out in the chicken.

The anterior wall can be anastomosed first if there is room to flip the double clamp. If not, the posterior wall can be completed through the anterior wall.

Advantages

- Quick technique.

- Less likely to bleed on clamp removal.

- If clamp space is tight, the posterior wall can be sutured through the front.

- Very good for anastomosing friable vessels.

Disadvantages

- Need to be accurate with suture placement and bite size.

- Correct horizontal tension is needed to avoid the 'purse-string' effect, particularly with veins.

- Have to be sure not to stitch in opposing wall.

- Not advisable without a double clamp.

It is advisable *not* to attempt this technique until you are experienced in interrupted suturing.

The anastomosis

Continuous sutures of 10/0 monofilament polyamide or monofilament polypropylene are used in all these exercises on rat femoral vessels (8/0 or 9/0 can be used for the chicken vessels).

Working on the anterior wall first is easier using the standard triangulation method, but if space is tight for flipping the clamp, then the posterior wall is anastomosed first through the anterior wall using the reverse triangulation technique.

DOI: 10.1201/9781003413080-12

The method shown throughout is the reverse triangulation to enhance the exercise difficulty (normal 120° triangulation technique suture placement can be used if vessel access is not a problem).

The idea is to place the first two stay sutures at 120° onto the posterior wall and apply horizontal tension. This flattens and stabilises the posterior wall so that the anterior 240° falls away from the posterior. With the correct tension, the anterior wall opens as a 'mouth' through which the posterior wall can be anastomosed (**Figure 12.1**).

Reverse triangulation technique

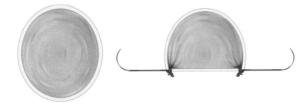

Figure 12.1 Placement of 120° stay sutures on *posterior* wall.

Femoral artery continuous anastomosis

● Clamp and prepare the artery (see Chapter 7) using the double clamps.

● Place the first stay suture (one double and two single throws) into the 120° point on the proximal and distal *posterior wall* on the left side. Leave the short end of the suture attached (**Figure 12.2**).

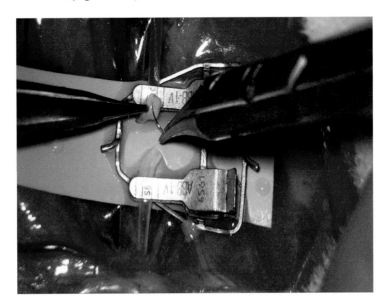

Figure 12.2 Placement of first stay suture.

- Place a second stay suture on the right hand side into the 120° point on the proximal and distal *posterior* wall.

- Leave the 'short' end long enough to fix to the right-hand cleat; the 'long' end has the needle attached (**Figure 12.3**).

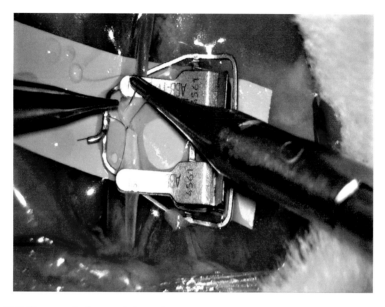

Figure 12.3 Placement of second stay suture.

- Place enough horizontal tension to straighten the posterior wall and open the anterior wall into a 'mouth' (**Figure 12.4**).

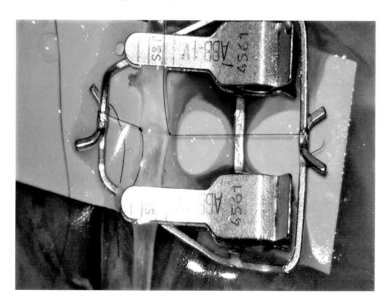

Figure 12.4 Anterior 'mouth'.

● Place the next stitch into the posterior wall as close to the stay suture as possible.

● Go from outside in on the proximal wall then direct the needle back out, then from outside in on the distal side (the needle should now be on the inside of the posterior wall) (**Figure 12.5**). This manoeuvre ensures the stitch is placed as close to the stay suture as possible and ensures a gap is not left in the distal posterior wall that could bleed.

● Gradually work along the posterior wall, taking 'arterial-size' bites, one needle-thickness apart.

● Adjust tension as you go but do not 'purse string'.

● Finish the last stitch as close to the left stay suture as possible. Tie with a double loop to the short end of the stay suture and keep the needle attached.

If the needle is kept to the left and the suture to the right, this minimises the risk of the suture tangling.

● Bring the needle through to the anterior wall and work along to the right-hand stay suture.

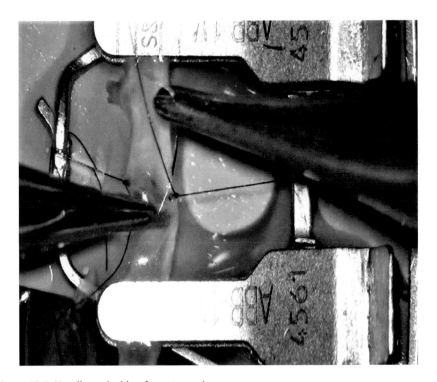

Figure 12.5 Needle on inside of anastomosis.

If the needle is kept to the right and the suture to the left this minimises the risk of the suture tangling on the posterior wall.

● Detach the stay suture from the cleat and tie with a double and two single throws (**Figure 12.6**).

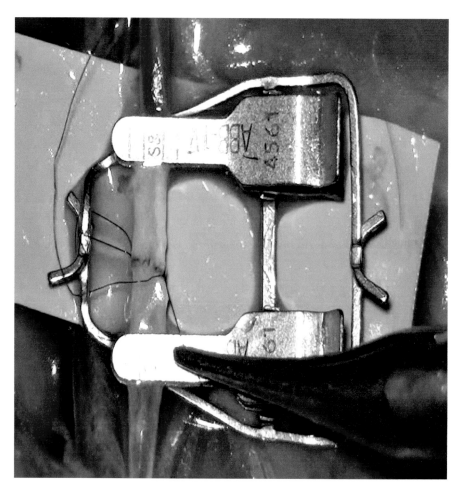

Figure 12.6 Detachment of the first stay suture.

Ensure you use a double throw; a single throw will not lock, and the artery will narrow.

● Remove the other stay suture.

● Remove the double clamp distal end first (**Figure 12.7**).

● Check flow with the 'milk' test.

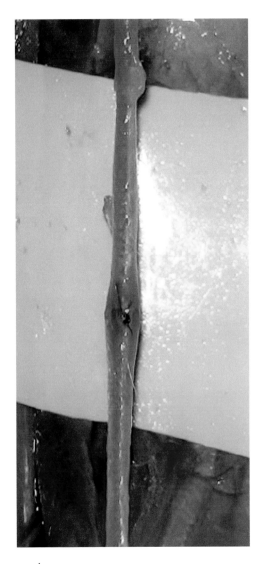

Figure 12.7 Clamp removal.

Femoral vein continuous anastomosis

This is performed in the same manner as the femoral artery.

- Clamp and prepare the vein (see Chapter 7) using the double clamps.

- Place the first stay suture (one double and two single throws) into the 120° point on the proximal and distal *posterior* wall on the left side.

- Attach the long end of the suture (with the needle) to the cleat and then cut.

- Leave the 'short' end of the suture ~5 mm long (**Figure 12.8**).

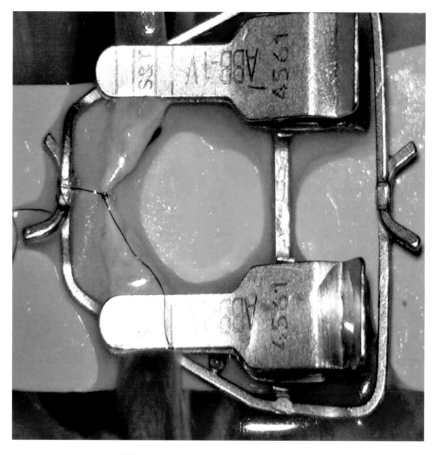

Figure 12.8 Attachment of first stay suture.

- Place the second stay suture on the right hand side into the 120° point on the proximal and distal *posterior* wall.

- Leave the 'short' end long enough to fix to the right-hand cleat.

- Place enough horizontal tension to straighten the posterior wall and open the anterior wall into a 'mouth' (**Figure 12.9**).

- Go from outside in on the proximal wall, then direct the needle back out and then from outside in on the distal side (the needle should now be on the inside of the posterior wall) (**Figure 12.10**). This prevents leaving a 'pouch' of vessel wall next to the stay stitch that may bleed.

- Place the next stitch into the posterior wall as close to the stay suture as possible.

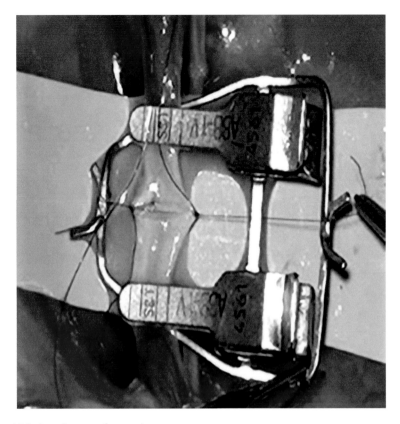

Figure 12.9 Attachment of second stay suture.

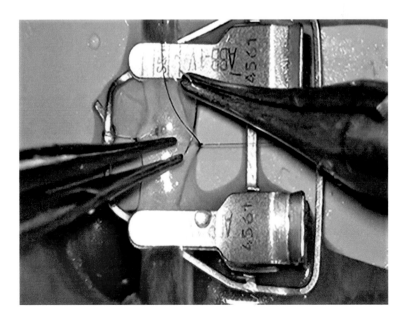

Figure 12.10 Needle on inside of anastomosis.

- Gradually work along the posterior wall, taking 'venous-size' bites, two needle-thicknesses apart.
- Adjust tension as you go but do not 'purse string'.

For very friable vessels, place two to three loops of stitch before adjusting tension, and this will negate vessel tears.

- When the posterior anastomosis is complete, take the needle back outside as close to the stay suture as possible.
- Tie the stitch to the 'short end' of the stay suture using a double throw (**Figure 12.11**).

This ensures that horizontal tension is kept.

Remember, if the needle is kept to the left and the suture to the right, this minimises the risk of the suture tangling.

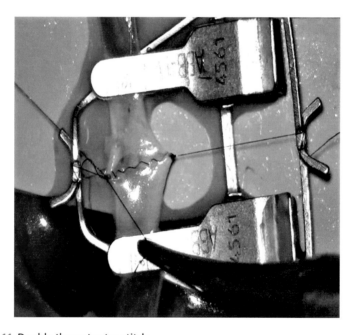

Figure 12.11 Double throw to stay stitch.

- Using the still attached needle, insert the next stitch into the anterior wall, ensuring it is as close to the stay suture as possible (**Figure 12.12**).
- Work along the anterior wall, adjusting the tension as you go and using the previous 'loop' as a stay suture (**Figure 12.13**).
- Finish the last stitch as close to the stay suture as possible.

Ensure the posterior wall is not caught as you stitch.

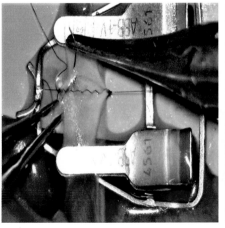 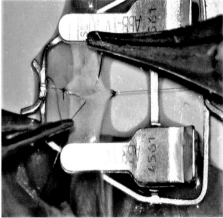

Figure 12.12 First stitch of anterior wall.

Figure 12.13 Using the previous 'loop' as stay stitch.

- Detach the stay suture from the cleat and tie with a double and two single throws – ensure you use a double throw; a single throw will not lock, and the vein will concertina and narrow.
- Remove the other stay suture.
- Remove the double clamp proximal end first (**Figure 12.14**).
- Check flow with the 'milk' test.

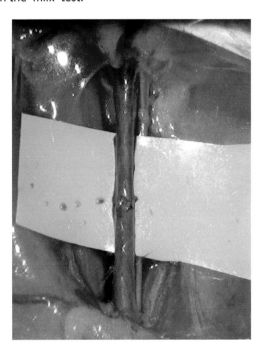

Figure 12.14 Clamp removal.

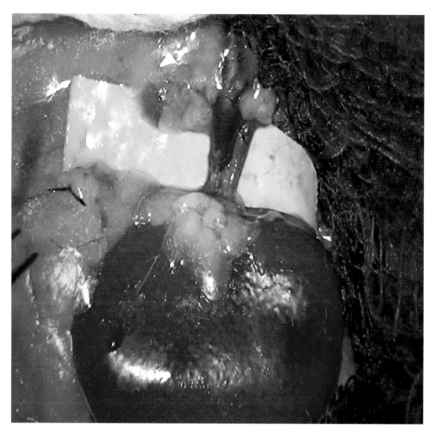

Figure 12.15 Renal vessels end-to-end continuous suturing.

For a more advanced exercise with this method, it can also be used for the end-to-end anastomosis of the renal vessels – see Chapter 13 for the renal harvest procedure. Instead of transecting the vessels at the junction of the aorta/vena cava, the renal vessels can be transected at the midpoint of their length and then anastomosed (**Figure 12.15**).

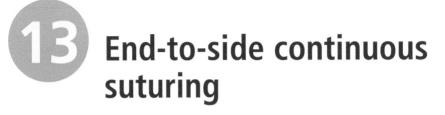

End-to-side continuous suturing

Renal model with end-to-side continuous suturing

In this exercise, the rat renal vessels are anastomosed with a continuous end-to-side suturing technique to the aorta and vena cava.

The harvest of the kidney tests dissection skills, as the renal vessels are delicate and intertwined and the dissection of the aorta and vena cava for the anastomoses has to be executed with great care. This also includes preparation of the optimal operative field and mimics the idea of a free flap using a continuous end-to-side suture technique.

The same exercise can also be executed with interrupted sutures if preferred (see Chapter 8).

This exercise can be mimicked in the chicken by utilising the end-to-side preparation of the vessels (see Chapter 8) but using the continuous suturing method described in the rat renal model.

This method shows anastomosis of the anterior walls first, but if access is an issue, then the posterior wall can be sutured through the anterior using the reverse 120° or triangulation technique described in Chapter 12.

The right kidney is used, as the pedicle will be much shorter and the exercise more challenging. For the first attempt, harvest the left kidney, as the left kidney has a longer pedicle.

Advantages:

● Quick technique.

● Less likely to bleed on clamp removal.

● If clamp space is tight, the posterior wall can be sutured through the front (reverse triangulation technique see Chapter 12).

● Very good for anastomosing friable vessels.

DOI: 10.1201/9781003413080-13

Disadvantages:

- Need to be accurate with suture placement and bite size.

- Correct horizontal tension is needed to avoid the 'purse-string' effect, particularly with veins.

- Have to be sure not to stitch the opposing wall.

It is advisable *not* to attempt this technique until you are experienced in interrupted suturing and have tried the end-to-end continuous exercise.

Renal exposure in the rat

- Using a No. 10 scalpel blade, a skin incision is made from the xiphisternum to just above the pubis.

- Using the scalpel tip, a small incision is made into the peritoneum along the linear alba, and this is extended using scissors.

- The peritoneum is retracted using four retractors.

- The bowel is wrapped in damp warm swabs and retracted to the left/right to give access to the left/right kidney – dissect the vessels right back to the aorta/ vena cava.

- A further damp swab is used to retract the stomach (left side) or liver (right side) as needed.

Renal harvest

- Using adventitia scissors and fine-toothed forceps, the fat around the kidney is cut free, taking care not to sever the renal pedicle or ureter (**Figure 13.1**).

- The renal artery and vein are carefully dissected from each other (the artery and vein can be entwined and multibranched) and freed down to the aorta/vena cava (**Figure 13.2**).

- The ureter is dissected free and a length of ~2 cm harvested.

- The kidney can be elevated using a damp swab to gain access to the posterior side of the vessels (**Figure 13.3**).

- The renal artery is tied off as close to the aorta as possible with 7/0 silk; it is then severed as close to the tie as possible.

- The renal vein is tied off as close to the vena cava as possible and transected.

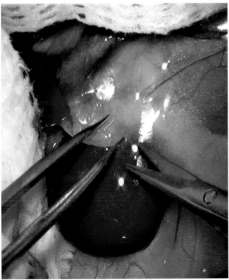 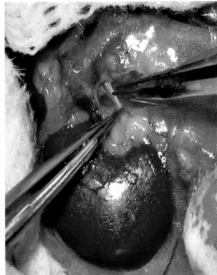

Figure 13.1 Freeing the fat capsule.   Figure 13.2 Vessel exposure.

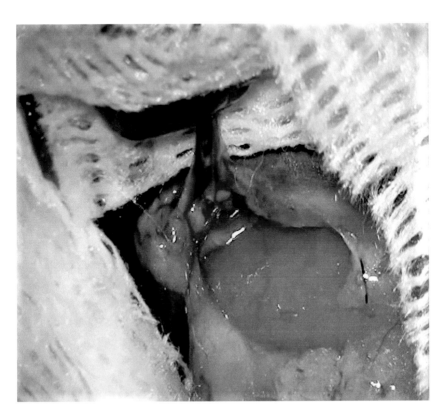

Figure 13.3 Posterior vessel dissection.

- The kidney is placed upright and is flushed with ~3 mL of heparinised saline through both the vein and the renal artery (in some cases, it may be necessary to flush two to three branches of the artery to ensure a clean flush) (**Figure 13.4**).

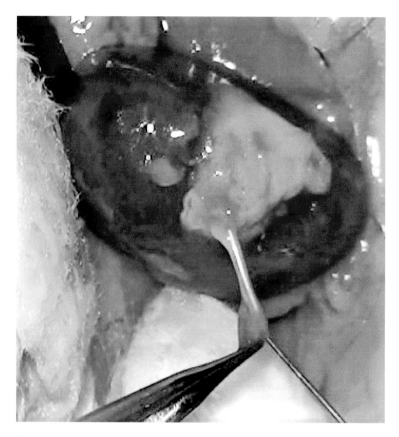

Figure 13.4 Renal perfusion.

The kidney can be placed into cold heparinised saline whilst the vena cava and aorta are dissected.

Aorta/vena cava vessel preparation

- The aorta/vena cava are dissected free for ~1 cm from the left renal vessels down to left iliolumbar vessels.
- Use blunt dissection with forceps to free the overlying fat.
- Swab sticks are a safe way to part excess fat from around the vessels (**Figure 13.5**).
- Side arms can be cauterised to free the vessels.

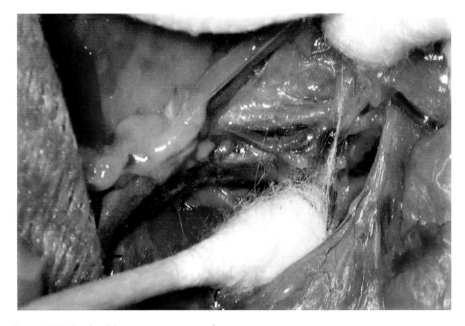

Figure 13.5 Swab sticks to remove excess fat.

The vena cava is friable, so take great care with the dissection (**Figure 13.6**).

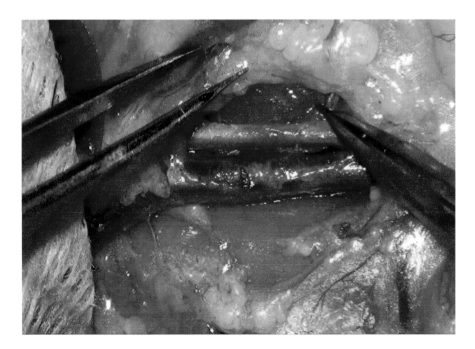

Figure 13.6 Completed dissection.

The anastomoses

Continuous sutures of 10/0 monofilament polyamide or monofilament polypropylene are used in all these exercises on rat renal vessels (8/0 or 9/0 can be used for the chicken vessels).

Venous anastomosis

- Place a background under the vena cava, and place single clamps at either end (distal first).

- Make a venotomy with Vannas scissors in the centre of the anterior wall (**Figure 13.7**).

- Flush and extend the venotomy to the outside diameter of the horizontally stretched renal vein.

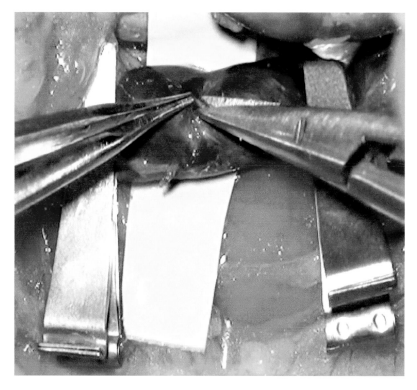

Figure 13.7 Venotomy.

- Position the kidney at a distance and place the first half of the suture at 180° into the renal vein.

- With a long length of free suture, place the second part of the stitch into the proximal end of the vena cava.

If the kidney is placed opposite the vena cava, it is very difficult to access the renal vein because of the angle caused by the underlying bowel.

Placing the stitch with the kidney at a distance makes suture placement easier – the kidney is then put in position and the stitch completed; this causes the renal vein to become extended from the kidney, making the second stitch much easier (**Figure 13.8**).

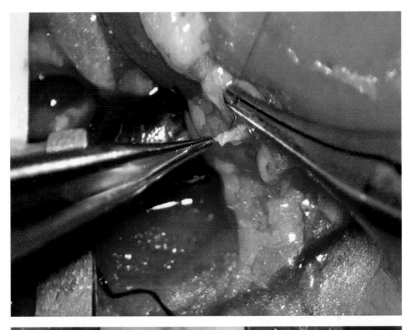

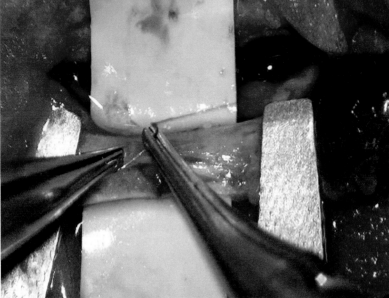

Figure 13.8 First stitch placement.

- Position the kidney to ensure there is no tension on the anastomosis.

  - The kidney can be secured in place with a damp swab.

- Secure the stitch with one double and two single throws (stay suture) and then cut the needle end of the suture free – leave the other end ~5 mm long.

- Place a second stay suture at 180° into the renal vein and vena cava – leave the needle end of the suture attached. Leave the other suture end ~5 mm long (**Figure 13.9**).

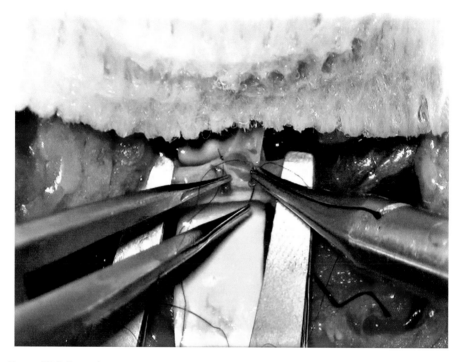

Figure 13.9 Second stay suture.

- On completion of the second stay suture, adjust the tension if necessary to clearly reveal the posterior wall.

- Place the next suture as close to the stay suture as possible.

- Place the first two running sutures into place *before* adjusting the tension to prevent tearing of the friable venous walls (**Figure 13.10**).

- Complete the stitch by tying to the ~5 mm long end with a *double*[1] throw and two single throws (**Figure 13.11**).

- Carefully reverse the kidney to expose the posterior venous wall.

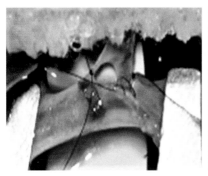

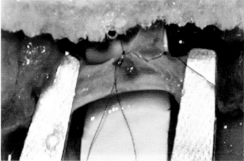

Figure 13.10 Adjusting tension.

Figure 13.11 Completed anterior wall.

- Place the next suture as close to the stay suture as possible.

- Place the first two running sutures into place *before* adjusting the tension to prevent tearing of the friable venous walls.

- Complete the stitch by tying to the ~5 mm long end with a *double* throw and two single throws as before (**Figure 13.12**).

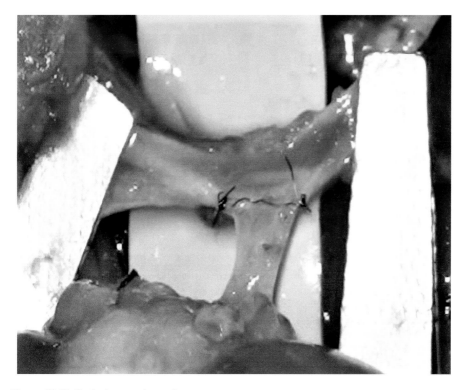

Figure 13.12 Posterior anastomosis.

Arterial anastomosis

● Place a background under the aorta and place single clamps at either end (proximal first).

● Clear the adventitia from the anterior wall with Vannas scissors.

● Make an arteriotomy with Vannas scissors in the centre of the anterior wall.

● Flush and extend the arteriotomy to the outside diameter of the horizontally stretched renal artery (**Figure 13.13**).

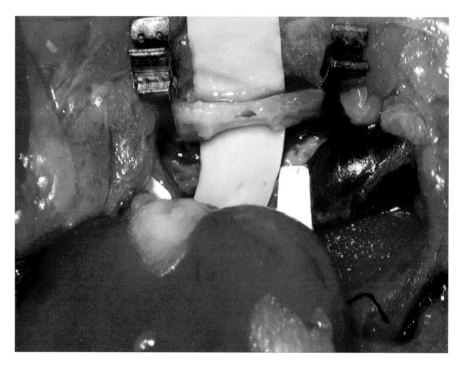

Figure 13.13 Arteriotomy.

● Secure the first stitch with a double and two single throws (stay suture) and then cut the needle end of the suture free – leave other end ~5 mm long.

● Place a second stay suture at 180° into the renal artery and aorta– leave the needle end of the suture attached. Leave the other suture end ~5 mm long.

● Place the next suture as close to the stay suture as possible then continue until the left hand stay suture is reached.

● Complete the stitch by tying to the ~5 mm long end with a *double* throw and two single throws as before (**Figure 13.14**).

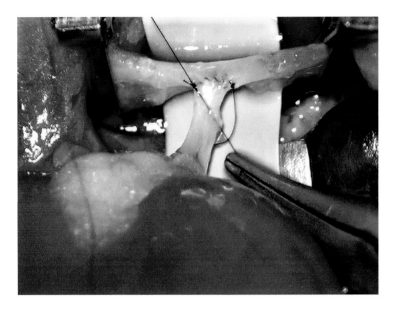

Figure 13.14 Anterior anastomosis.

- Carefully reverse the kidney to expose the posterior arterial wall.

- Place the next suture as close to the stay suture as possible then continue until the right hand stay suture is reached.

- Complete the stitch by tying to the ~5 mm long end with a *double* throw and two single throws as before (**Figure 13.15**).

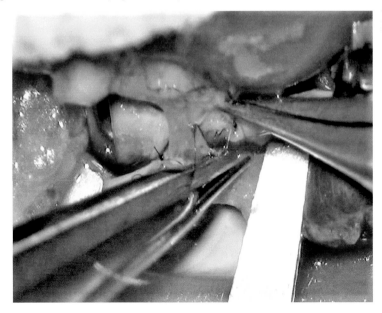

Figure 13.15 Posterior anastomosis.

Spot the deliberate mistake! The venotomy and arteriotomy have been performed too close together, making the arterial anastomosis more difficult. So beware! Venotomy is more proximal and arteriotomy is more distal!

Clamp removal

Remove the venous clamps proximal first and then remove the arterial clamps distal first.

Apply a damp swab until the oozing stops and then place the kidney into position (**Figure 13.16**).

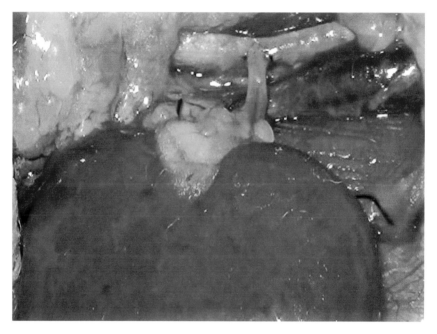

Figure 13.16 Reperfused kidney.

If the kidney remains pale, check arterial anastomosis. If congestion occurs, check venous anastomosis.

Note

1 Ensure a double throw to ensure the stitch locks. If not, the vein tension will be compromised and lead to narrowing of the vessel and ultimately anastomotic failure.

14 Peripheral nerve repair

General notes

Each trunk of a peripheral nerve comprises groups of nerve fibres gathered together into bundles termed fascicles. The nerve trunk is invested in loose epineurium, whilst each fascicle is surrounded by perineurium. It is really impossible to differentiate between sensory and motor fascicles, as they are each made up of a mixture of sensory, motor and sympathetic nerve fibres (**Figure 14.1**).

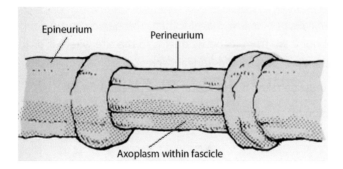

Figure 14.1 Peripheral nerve.

It is possible to repair peripheral nerves by suturing together the epineurium, the perineurium or a combination of the two. The most commonly used is epineural repair. Sutures (9/0 or 10/0) on cutting needles have been designed for this task.

Whatever the method of anastomosis, the surgeon must seek close apposition of fascicles with blood vessels aligned and complete reduction of torque (i.e., longitudinal twist) and tension. Tension is the most common cause of failure, as it inhibits the vascular supply to the nerve and increases the influx of fibrocytes.

Nerve model

The largest available nerve to anastomose in the rat is the sciatic nerve – this nerve is not a good model for a human nerve, as it is friable, but does give an indication of how to suture a nerve.

The chicken nerve is larger and more robust and is a better model for the human nerve – dissection is the same as for vascular access.

DOI: 10.1201/9781003413080-14

Rat sciatic nerve

Exposure

- With a scalpel, a 3 cm-long skin incision is made running parallel with the junction of the biceps femoris and the gluteus maximus muscles.

- Using bow scissors, the skin is bluntly dissected from the underlying muscles and is then retracted.

- Separate but do not cut the muscles and divide adherent tissue by blunt dissection, taking care not to rupture the superior gluteal or the medial femoral circumflex vessels.

- The sciatic nerve now lies to the right covered by the biceps femoris muscle and can be visualised once the gluteus maximus and biceps femoris muscles have been retracted with either a Jenson's retractor or paper clips attached to rubber bands (**Figure 14.2**).

- Using the microscope at low magnification, the nerve can be gently freed for a length of about 2 cm from its pelvic origins to the site where it divides into three branches (the tibial, sural and peroneal nerves).

- Great care must be taken not to rupture the epineural sheath.

- To take tension off the nerve, unpin the rat leg and tape it to the tail.

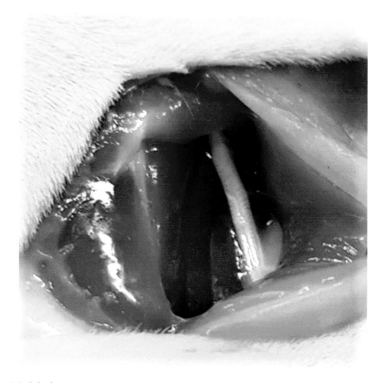

Figure 14.2 Sciatic exposure.

Epineural repair

This described repair of a rat nerve consists of approximately nine sutures joining the epineural connective tissue investing the nerve trunk (a chicken nerve would take approximately six to ten sutures, and a human nerve of this size is more robust and would take approximately four sutures).

- The nerve is dissected free from the surrounding tissue using sharp dissection. Blunt dissection can rupture the fragile epineural layer.

- Background material should be placed under the nerve and the field irrigated (**Figure 14.3**).

- Under low magnification, the nerve is sharply transected, preferably with a diamond or ruby scalpel. Scissors tend to compress the nerve but have been used here as other instruments may not be available.

- The divided nerve will retract a considerable distance, so it may be necessary to move the rat's leg slightly to allow coaptation without tension (**Figure 14.4**).

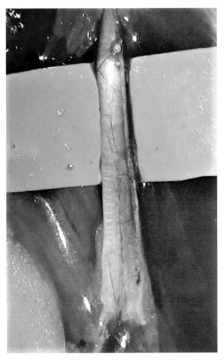 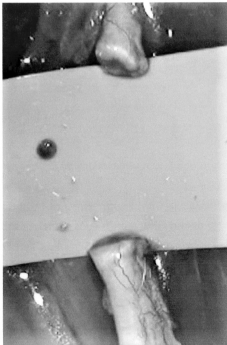

Figure 14.3 Nerve dissection.   Figure 14.4 Tension release.

When the nerve ends are examined under high power, you will usually find that the sciatic nerve of rats is divided into three fascicles. It is important to align the proximal and distal nerve segments so that the fascicles are matched in their correct rotation, using the angle of incision, the size and grouping of the fascicles and the epineural vascular topography as visual guides to matching.

The epineurium should not be stripped from the nerve segments, as this is important to the vascular supply of the anastomosed nerve.

- Grasp the epifascicular epineurium with forceps working under 6–10× magnification and pass a 9/0 or 10/0 suture at the 120° position. Take 1 mm bites out of the epineurium and pass the needle so that it lies parallel with the surface just beneath the epineurium, not into the perineurium, and taking care not to transfix any of the fascicles.

- Secure with a double and two single throws, leaving the proximal end long. Repeat at the opposite 120° point (**Figure 14.5**).

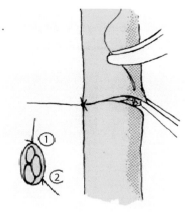

Figure 14.5 Stay suture placement.

- Place the third and fourth sutures between the two stays, tying a simple square knot and cutting both ends short. All subsequent sutures should be simple square knots (**Figure 14.6**).

- The nerve is now rotated about its longitudinal axis using the stay sutures, the long ends of which are attached to single Acland clamps to hold the nerve in position (**Figure 14.7**).

Before suturing the posterior wall, attention must be paid to the axoplasm. Unlike human nerves, the axoplasm is exuded continuously from the proximal nerve stump and can make the anastomosis difficult to complete. To alleviate this, a few millimetres of the proximal and distal axoplasm are resected, creating an empty epineural 'pocket' in which to place the exuding proximal axoplasm. This is not necessary in humans, as the axoplasm does not protrude.

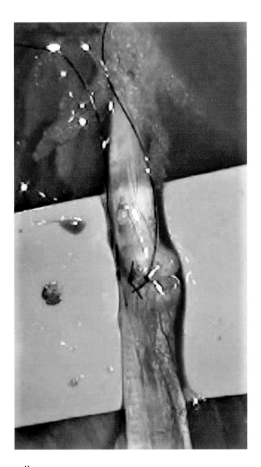

Figure 14.6 Anterior wall.

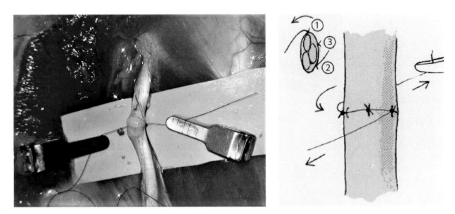

Figure 14.7 Posterior wall.

Care should be taken when tying subsequent sutures that the epineural walls are brought together without involving the neuroplasm. This should be gently 'tucked' into the distal pocket as the stitches are brought together.

● The fifth suture is placed at the midpoint position and the proximal end left long.

● The single clamp is removed and placed onto this midpoint suture to ensure tension; this rotates the nerve and allows placement of the sixth and seventh sutures (**Figure 14.8**).

● The Acland clamp is then moved to the left, still attached to the midpoint suture; this then rotates the nerve to the left and allows placement of the eighth and ninth sutures (**Figure 14.9**).

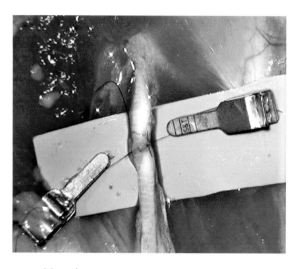

Figure 14.8 Clamp repositioned.

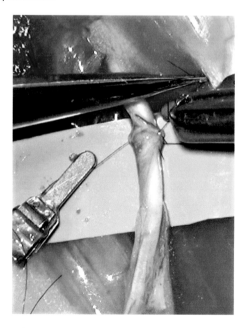

Figure 14.9 Nerve rotated.

Once the anastomosis is complete, the Acland clamps are removed and the nerve rotated to its original position. The stay sutures are then cut short, the background material removed and the area irrigated (**Figure 14.10**).

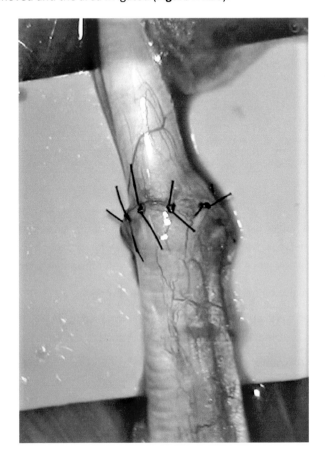

Figure 14.10 Completed nerve anastomosis.

Interpositional nerve grafts

To mimic the clinical situation in which interpositional nerve grafts are used to join damaged nerves without undue tension, the rat sciatic nerve is removed from one leg via the standard surgical approach and grafted onto the opposite limb.

It is possible to harvest between 1.0 and 1.2 cm of donor nerve. With the chicken nerve, 1 cm can be removed, reversed and then anastomosed into the gap.

● Excise 0.5 cm of nerve from the recipient side. The nerve stumps will spring back and create a gap to be bridged of at least 1.0 cm.

● The graft is then sutured in position using the standard epineural anastomosis described earlier (**Figure 14.11**).

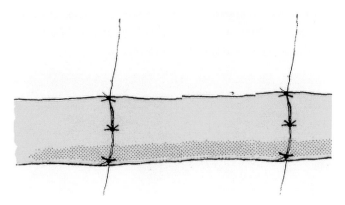

Figure 14.11 Nerve graft.

Interfasicular repair

This repair is no longer used in the clinical situation due to excessive fibrosis occurring within the nerve; however, it is a useful exercise for dissection and anastomotic purposes, particularly when wanting to repair nerves at the supramicrosurgical level.

This exercise can also be performed using the chicken nerve.

● The sciatic nerve is exposed and dissected clear for a sufficient length to allow transection 5 mm proximal to its division into tibial, sural and peroneal nerves.

● Using the microscope at 10× magnification, dissect and roll back the peripheral epineurium for a distance of about 1 mm, then separate each fascicle gently, teasing apart the interfascicular epineurium.

● Transect each fascicle.

It is possible to place two sutures 180° apart in the two smaller fascicles, passing the needle (9/0 or 10/0) through the perineurium only. In the larger fascicle, it may be possible to place three sutures (**Figure 14.12**).

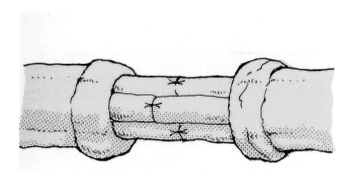

Figure 14.12 Fascicular anastomosis.

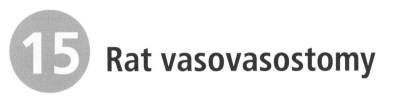

15 Rat vasovasostomy

This exercise utilises rat testes and the vas anastomosed end to end using a two-layer technique. The same exercise could be carried out on abattoir specimens obtainable from farm animals if available.

Vasovasostomy can be performed in rats as a model for training and research, although the rat vas lacks the thick musculature characteristics of the human vas.

In man, the vasovasostomy can also be completed either by a single layer of interrupted sutures through the whole wall of the vas or by two layers of sutures, one joining mucosa to mucosa and the other seromusculature to seromusculature.

The suture used throughout is a 10/0 nylon for the rat and in man 9/0 nylon on a micropoint needle.

The method described is the modified two-layer technique, though other techniques are described in the literature.

Vasovasostomy clamps

When attempting a vasovasostomy, it is best to use specially designed double clamps; these will make the operation that much easier but are expensive to purchase (**Figure 15.1**).

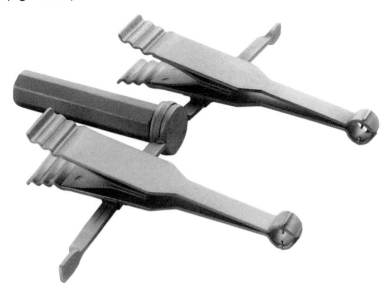

Figure 15.1 Vasovasostomy clamps.

DOI: 10.1201/9781003413080-15

Advantages:

- Reduces operating time
- Ends clamp slippage with the use of flat-tipped, non-penetrating steel spikes
- Gentle to mucosa
- Two-directional fold that facilitates anterior and posterior wall anastomosis
- Adjustable and lockable
- Easily stabilised by attaching a haemostat

The vasovasostomy described in the rat utilises two single clamps instead of the approximator clamp, as some units may not have them due to availability or cost.

Rat dissection

A vertical incision over the scrotum is carefully deepened until the testis, epididymis and straight portion of the vas are revealed. The whole structure is elevated and placed onto a damp swab to hold it in position (**Figure 15.2**).

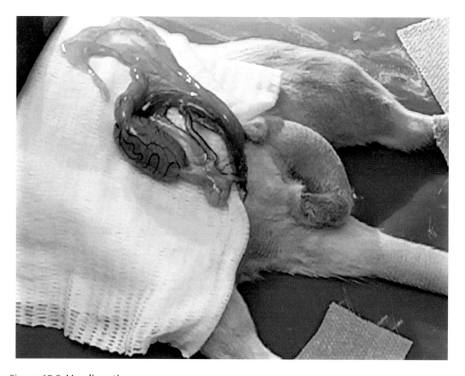

Figure 15.2 Vas dissection.

Exposing the whole length of the vas gives room for practising multiple anastomoses (**Figure 15.3**).

Anatomy

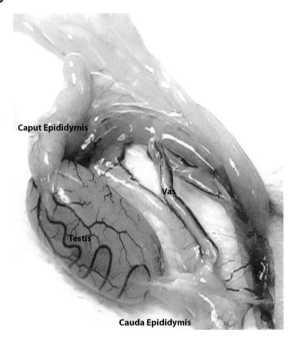

Figure 15.3 Anatomy.

Vasovasostomy: Two-layer method

There are a few different techniques described in the literature; the most common is the two-layer or modified two-layer method. Either method can be used for practice; the method used here for training purposes is the modified two layer. This differs from the standard two layer, as the first two or three stitches are placed through the full thickness of the vas deferens, not just the mucosal layer.

Vasovasostomy modified two-layer method

With this method, four (in the rat) to six (in man) sutures are placed through the full thickness of the vas. These sutures ensure that the lumens on both sides of the vas are correctly aligned.

Stitches are then placed in the outer layer of the two ends to prevent sperm leakage and potential scarring or breakdown.

The thick walls of the vas can prevent adequate alignment if anastomosed by the seromuscular layer alone.

Vasovasostomy preparation

It is important that the area is kept irrigated throughout the procedure to alleviate dehiscence and to prevent later adhesions.

- The adventitia is gently freed from around the vas (**Figure 15.4**).

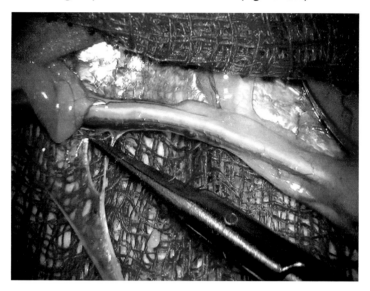

Figure 15.4 Adventitia removal.

- The main vessel (artery of the vas deferens) underlying the vas is carefully dissected free and preserved (**Figure 15.5**).

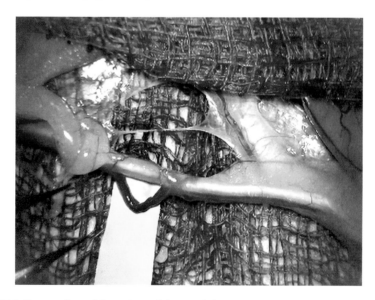

Figure 15.5 Preservation of the artery of the vas deferens.

It is important that before the vas is divided any possible bleeding is controlled, as any oozing will obscure the transected end of the vas and make anastomosis more difficult.

- The smaller vessel can also be dissected free and preserved (in man) or be ligated or cauterised in the rat model.

- Once the possibility of any bleeding is alleviated, the vas can be placed over a piece of background material and then divided.

- The first suture is placed at the 10 o'clock position through the seromuscular layer and into the lumen on both sides, leaving the stitch *untied* until the 2 o'clock suture is in position (**Figure 15.6**).

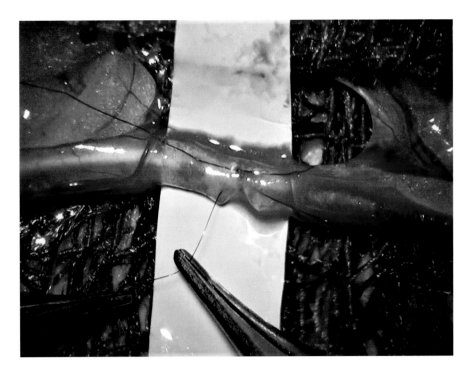

Figure 15.6 First stitch placement.

- Once in position, the stitches are tied and cut.
  - Due to the thickness of the vas wall, the stitches should consist of a double throw followed by two single throws.
- The ends of the vas are again aligned with two 10/0 sutures, this time through the seromuscular layer at 180°. These are secured, leaving one end of the stitch long in each case. These help to manipulate the vessel and place subsequent sutures.

- The next stitch is placed equidistant to these two on the anterior wall and the gaps between filled with two to three more stitches (**Figure 15.7**).

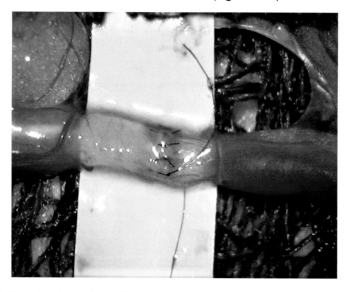

Figure 15.7 Completed anterior wall.

- On completion of the anterior wall, the vas is flipped over (this is easy if a double clamp is used), or alternatively, if this clamp is not available, single clamps can be applied to the long suture ends. These act as weights and help to keep the vas in place for the posterior anastomosis (**Figure 15.8**).

- As before, two sutures are placed at 10 o'clock and 2 o'clock into the vas lumen and not tied until both are in place.

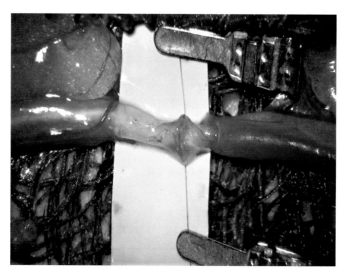

Figure 15.8 Posterior wall exposure.

- The next stitch is placed in the middle of the posterior wall into the seromuscular layer, leaving one end long. Another one to two sutures are placed alongside this.

- To reach the last quadrant, a single clamp can be removed and placed onto the central posterior stitch. This rotates the vas and makes it easier to place the last one to two sutures (**Figure 15.9**).

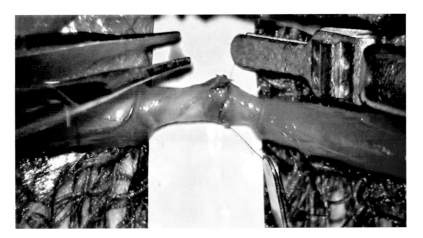

Figure 15.9 Rotating to stitch the last quadrant.

- On completion, make sure the vas is not twisted and remove the background material (**Figure 15.10**).

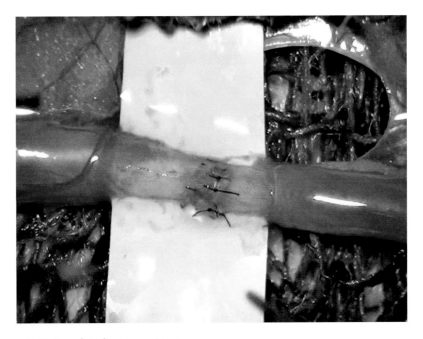

Figure 15.10 Completed vasovasostomy.

16 Rat epididymovasostomy

The initial dissection is the same as the for the vasovasostomy. The suture used throughout is 10/0 nylon for the rat and 9/0 for man on a micropoint needle.

Double-armed needles are available that make the anastomosis much easier but are expensive, so for practice purposes and as some units do not have access to them, single needles are utilised.

In this module the exercise utilises rat testes and the vas is anastomosed using an intussusception two-suture transverse technique (modified for practice in the rat).

Epididymovasostomy clamps

When attempting an epididymovasostomy, it is best to use specially designed double clamps; as mentioned, these will make the operation that much easier but are expensive to purchase (**Figure 16.1**).

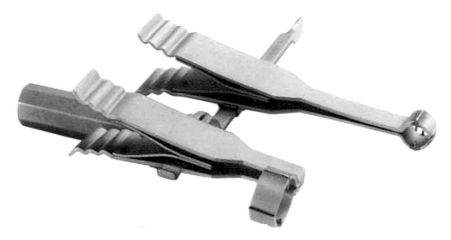

Figure 16.1 Epididymovasostomy clamp example.

Advantages:

- Reduces operating time
- Ends clamp slippage with the use of flat-tipped, non-penetrating steel spikes
- Gentle to mucosa

DOI: 10.1201/9781003413080-16

- Two-directional fold that facilitates anterior and posterior wall anastomosis

- Adjustable and lockable

- Easily stabilised by attaching a haemostat

The epididymovasostomy described here in the rat does not use these clamps, as some units may not have them due to availability or cost.

Various methods are described in the literature, and any of these could be used for training purposes. The method utilised for this exercise is an intussusception two-suture transverse technique. The transverse technique has been chosen, as the epididymis transection is easier to perform on the rat than with a longitudinal incision.

Epididymovasostomy dissection

Normally in man the caput epididymis is used, but in the rat exercise, the cauda is utilised, as the caput is too fragile (**Figure 16.2**).

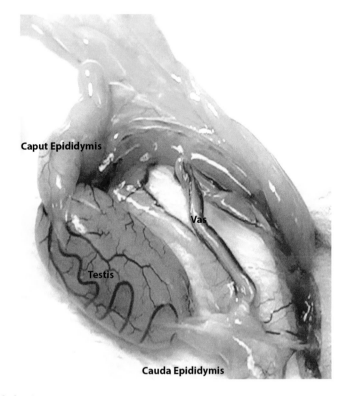

Figure 16.2 Anatomy.

It is important that the area is kept irrigated throughout the procedure to alleviate dehiscence and to prevent later adhesions.

● The adventitia is gently freed from around the vas (**Figure 16.3**).

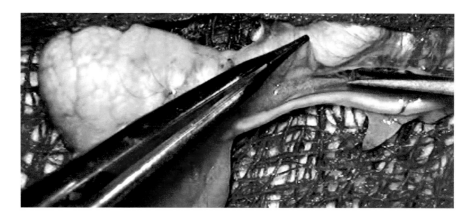

Figure 16.3 Adventitia removal.

● The main vessel underlying the vas can be carefully dissected free, doubly ligated and cut (**Figure 16.4**).

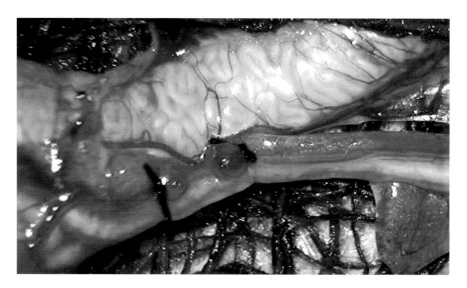

Figure 16.4 Dividing the artery of the vas deferens.

● It is important that before the vas is divided any possible bleeding is controlled, as any oozing will obscure the transected end of the vas and make anastomosis more difficult.

The vas is then transected, leaving a longer 'stump' on the vas side (**Figure 16.5**).

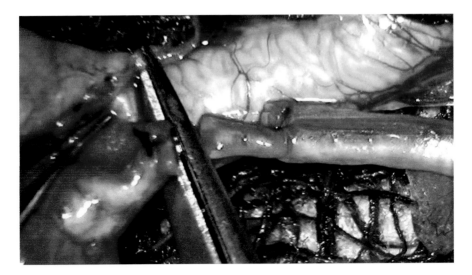

Figure 16.5 Dividing the vas.

- The vas is then placed adjacent to the cauda.

- With scissors, an incision is made in the caudal sac equal to the outside diameter of the vas (**Figure 16.6**).

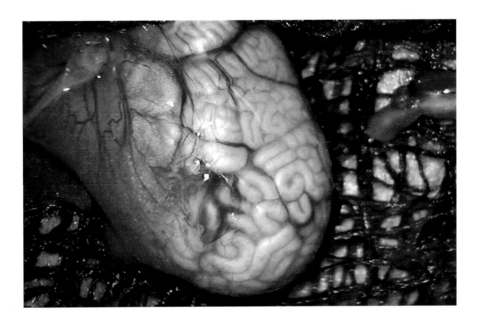

Figure 16.6 Incising the caudal sac.

● The epididymis tubule is *gently* freed by blunt dissection (in man, sharp dissection is needed, as the tissue is much tougher) (**Figure 16.7**).

● Two 8/0 monofilament nylon sutures are placed on either side of the vas lumen and tied to secure the vas in place, ensuring there is no tension (**Figure 16.8**).

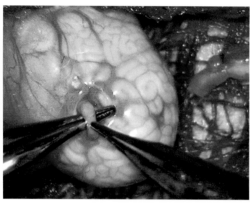

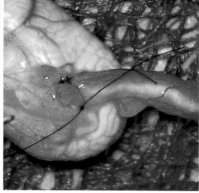

Figure 16.7 Exposing the tubule.   Figure 16.8 Securing with 8/0.

● The end of the vas is then resected to healthy, vascularised tissue and the vas lumen exposed (**Figure 16.9**).

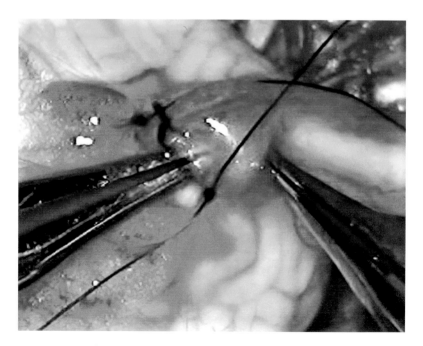

Figure 16.9 Exposing the vas lumen.

● Insert one 10/0 suture ~3 mm from the vas end from outside of the vas to the inside. Bring the needle through to the external vas opening and then transversely into the tubule. Leave the suture untied. Repeat for the other side (**Figure 16.10**).[1]

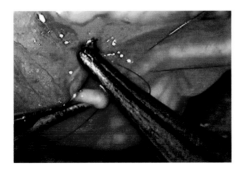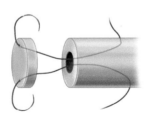

Figure 16.10 Insertion of first two sutures.

● Transversely, incise the tubule between the sutures with Vannas scissors, making the smallest cut possible (**Figure 16.11**).

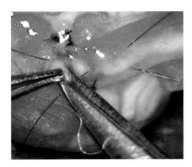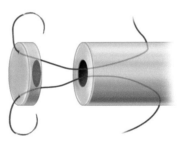

Figure 16.11 Incising the tubule transversely.

● Take the needles back into the vas and exit at the original entrance point. Double-tie each stitch, ensuring the tubule is invaginated into the vas (**Figure 16.12**).

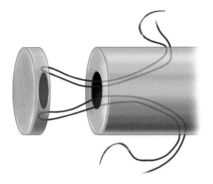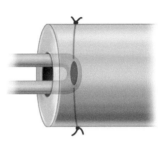

Figure 16.12 Invaginating the tubule.

● With 10/0 sutures placed into the vas muscularis, secure the vas to the caudal sac along the anterior wall (**Figure 16.13**).

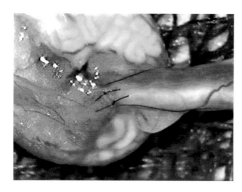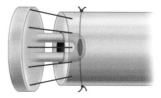

Figure 16.13 Securing the vas muscularis on the anterior wall.

● Complete the posterior wall with 10/0 interrupted sutures to secure the vas to the caudal sac.

● Position the vas so there is no tension present (**Figure 16.14**).

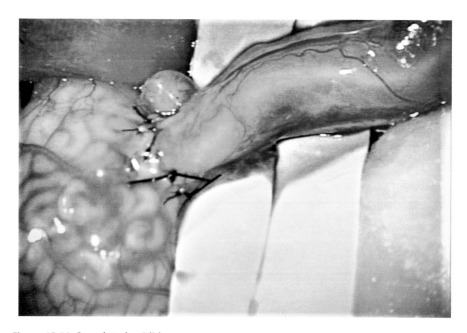

Figure 16.14 Completed epididymovasostomy.

Note

1 In man, the suture is normally placed into tubule first and then out through the vas. This puts unnecessary strain on a rat tubule, so the preference is to do it the other way a round.

17 Clinical practice

Key points:

- Properly maintained instruments are critical to success.

- Microvascular transfer has major surgical stress to the patient. Perioperative assessment is important.

- High blood flow into and out of the free tissue transfer is the key to success. Vessel selection is critical in ensuring success. When possible, use large-calibre vessels.

- Setting up the position of the microscope and the ergonomics of the chair are important.

- Postoperative support for blood pressure, intravascular volume and cardiac support is important in maintaining good flow through the free tissue transfer.

- The rate of successful salvage is inversely proportional to the elapsed time between the onset of ischaemia and clinical recognition. Postoperative monitoring is an essential element of microsurgery.

Preoperative

Free tissue transfer is a major surgical procedure, with significant surgical stress. Fluid loss, hypothermia and length of procedure all have significant effects on success. Patients must be critically assessed for cardiac, pulmonary and renal status and optimised.

Microsurgical instruments

Operating microscope

The operating microscope should have good optics, a wide field of view with a good depth and a strong light source. Other desirable features include binocular tube assemblies with an adjustable angle of inclination, an X-Y unit with a wide range of movement in both planes and independent focus and zoom controls for the surgeon and the assistant. An additional useful feature is an attached video camera that allows the scrub nurses and other surgical team members to view the anastomoses for teaching and training.

DOI: 10.1201/9781003413080-17

Instruments

Forceps, needle holders and scissors need to be well maintained. The forceps, which evolved from basic jeweller's tweezers, is the primary microsurgical instrument. The forceps are used to grasp tissue, manipulate and tie sutures and hold open a vascular lumen for suture placement. It is essential that the tips be smooth and without irregularity when scrutinised under the microscope.

Microsurgical needle holders must be designed so that they can firmly hold a needle without bending it or allowing it to slip. The jaws must be small so that they do not obstruct the field of view, and they must have a smooth surface so that they can grip the suture material. A round handle is particularly well suited to the rotations necessary for the precise placement of sutures.

Microvascular clamps are available as single clamps, which can be straight or angled, or as double-approximating clamps. Most clamps have nonslip surfaces to help grip the vessels when low-spring pressures is used. Generally, the smallest clamp that will hold a vessel without slipping should be chosen.

Nylon remains the most popular suture material for microsutures. Microsutures are available in sizes from 8-0 to 12-0. The most commonly used needles in microsurgery are between 75 and 100 microns in diameter. The needle may be cutting, tapered or a combination. Cutting needles are used to penetrate rigid tissues and are useful in nerve surgery and in ophthalmic surgery. Tapered-tip needles have a cone-shaped configuration with a sharp point and are designed to penetrate soft tissues with the smallest hole possible. Tapered-tip needles are usually used for microvascular anastomosis.

Intraoperative

Vessels

The key factor in achieving high reliability of free tissue transfer is to have a high rate of blood flow into and out of the flap. Therefore recipient vessel selection is one of the most critical steps in ensuring success. When possible, use large recipient vessels. When selecting donor vessels, it is better to select a vessel with a diameter of similar size to the flap vessels rather than attempt modifications.

Various factors must be considered when selecting the recipient vessels. The location of the defect has a great impact on the decision-making process. The particular flap that is selected determines the calibre and length of the donor vessels and thus affects the choice of recipient vessels. Prior radiation therapy and atherosclerosis of vessels in the region may also limit recipient vessel availability.

Selecting and isolating the recipient vessels before the flap pedicle is divided at the donor site is best. Additional time spent on recipient vessel preparation after the pedicle has been divided prolongs the ischaemic period of the flap unnecessarily. The vessels are isolated with vessel loops, which serve a dual purpose of obtaining proximal and distal control of the vessels and of elevating the vessels to an optimal position for microvascular anastomosis. Both the artery and vein should be dissected for a suitable length so that each anastomosis can be performed with good exposure. The recipient artery is divided and assessed for flow. Once adequate flow is demonstrated, a microvascular clamp is placed on the artery.

Vein grafts

In certain instances it is necessary to use vein grafts to prevent tension on an anastomosis or to bridge long gaps in regions with limited anatomical access.

Vein grafts can be harvested from virtually any location but are generally obtained from the upper or lower extremities. However, it is often more convenient to harvest a vein near the operative site. Another vein graft source is the cephalic vein, found in the deltopectoral groove.

Setting up for the anastomoses

Proper setup for the anastomoses is one of the most critical steps in a microsurgical procedure. When properly set up, the anastomoses are often easy to perform, with an economy of movement. A frequent error committed by less experienced surgeons is not spending enough time on this step.

- The optimal position should be achieved by the surgeons to accommodate comfortable elbow placement and movements of the wrists for ease of suturing.

- The surgeon's head and neck should be positioned comfortably when looking into the eyepieces of the microscope to minimise strain on the neck.

- The operative area should be clean and free of unnecessary instruments and sponges, and all things needed during the microvascular anastomoses, including a moist pad for cleaning the instruments, heparinised irrigation solution, microsurgical instruments and sutures, should be set up before the anastomoses are started.

- Optimal exposure of the vessels must be achieved. Good lighting is critical because it increases visual acuity and depth of field.

- The plane of each vessel should also be level. When the plane is uneven, this can result in focusing problems due to the limited depth of field that exists under high-power magnification.

A solid-coloured background may be placed under the vessels to visually simplify the area surrounding them and provide a smooth surface against which to suture. Unfavourable exposure of the vessels is responsible for many of the technical errors made during surgery. Therefore, gaining adequate exposure and taking the time to set up the vessels properly before performing the anastomoses is important.

Vessel preparation

The final preparation of both the recipient and donor vessels should be done under the operating microscope. The excess adventitia is trimmed from the end of each vessel so that it cannot become trapped in the lumen during the anastomosis. It is not necessary or desirable to dissect the adventitia past the distance that ensures a clean anastomosis. The lumen of each vessel is also inspected by turning up the end and peering directly into it under the microscope. Gentle irrigation is used to wash away any loose clots in the lumen.

The arterial intima may contain atheromatous plaques, in which case it is prudent to resect the vessel further to a section of lumen that is smooth. The vessel end may also be dilated gently with vessel-dilating forceps. Excessive stretching of a vessel, however, may result in intimal damage.

Suturing

Successful anastomosis requires an understanding of the physiological factors that affect anastomotic patency, technical competence and sound clinical judgment gained from experience.

In general, two surgeons participate in the microvascular anastomoses. Heparinised Ringer's lactate solution in a small syringe with a fine-gauge, blunt-tip needle is used to irrigate the lumen of each vessel. The assistant stabilises the vessel with forceps, irrigates the lumen to remove foreign material and assists in providing exposure so that the surgeon can place the sutures for anastomosis.

Either the artery or the vein may be anastomosed first. Flow to the flap does not have to be restored until both anastomoses are complete.

- You should place full-thickness sutures an appropriate distance from the vessel edge, as well as from one another, and tie them with the appropriate amount of tension.

- Partial-thickness sutures result in exposure of thrombogenic subintimal tissues.

In general, one should select the bite size that will achieve a reasonably watertight anastomosis with as few sutures as possible. Suture tension is also critical. Sutures tied too tightly can cause necrosis of a portion of the vessel wall, whereas sutures tied too loosely can result in exposure of thrombogenic subintimal tissue.

Poor technique can also contribute to anastomotic failure in other ways. Extra needle holes as a result of multiple attempts to pass the needle create sites for platelet plugs to form. Sutures passed obliquely through the vessel wall have a tendency to cut through the vessel wall when tied.

Suturing can be done using an interrupted or continuous suture technique. For small vessels, the interrupted technique is more precise. The continuous technique is faster but requires careful attention to the spacing of and the amount of tension on the sutures. Excessive tension tends to have a purse-string effect on an anastomosis, whereas insufficient tension tends to result in leaks between the sutures.

An anastomosis performed with couplers is a reliable alternative method of anastomosis and can be done for veins currently.

A coupler device, where the vessel ends are passed through opposing rings and everted on pins, approximates the rings which stay in place (**Figure 17.1**). These have an equivalent patency rate and do speed up venous anastomosis.

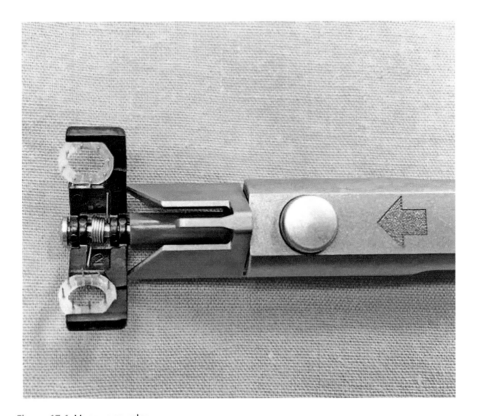

Figure 17.1 Venous coupler.

Patency tests

After flow is restored (**Figure 17.2**), the anastomoses are inspected for leaks. Large leaks need additional suturing, but small leaks will stop spontaneously.

Anastomotic patency can be assessed:

- Indirectly by observing the colour and the amount of bleeding from the dermis of the flap or its muscle tissue. Blood from the dermal edges of the flap should be bright red when the dermis is rubbed with a gauze sponge. Sluggish flow of blood is suggestive of an arterial problem. Rapid, profuse flow of dark blood indicates venous obstruction. Muscle flaps without skin islands should remain moist and reddish-pink during the insetting.

- Directly with a 'milking' test, which can be done on the vein by occluding flow just beyond the anastomosis with a forceps and milking the vessel distally with a second forceps until an empty segment of vessel is created. When the proximal forceps is released, brisk flow should be observed, with quick filling of the empty segment. Slow flow with poor distention of the vessel is suggestive of an anastomotic problem.

  - Where there remains any question about the patency of an anastomosis, the anastomosis should be partially or completely taken down and the lumen inspected.

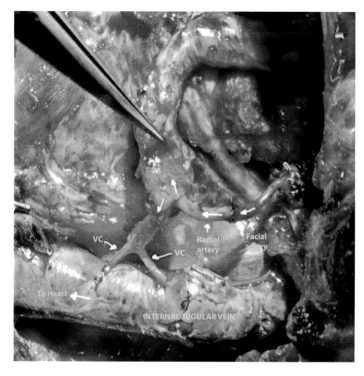

Figure 17.2 Radial artery and vena comitans anastomosis.

Postoperative monitoring

The rate of successful flap salvage has been shown to be inversely proportional to the elapsed time between the onset of ischaemia and its clinical recognition. For this reason, postoperative monitoring is an essential element of successful microsurgery.

- Hourly observation of the flap by trained personnel for the first several days is still considered the best means of postoperative monitoring.

- A pale flap with poor capillary refill usually indicates an arterial inflow problem, and a blue flap with a rapid refill indicates venous obstruction. Muscle flaps that have an arterial problem look dry and flaccid, while muscle flaps with venous obstruction appear dark and swollen.

- In addition, the flap can be pricked with a 20-gauge needle away from the pedicle and the quality of the bleeding observed. Bright red blood that appears right away and continues to form after being wiped away is a sign that all is well. No blood flow or serum ooze indicates arterial obstruction, and dark, rapid bleeding indicates venous obstruction. If there is any doubt, it is best to return to the operating room and explore the anastomosis.

In addition to monitoring flap colour, capillary refill and temperature, you can also monitor the flap with a handheld Doppler or a thermal camera.

Another option is the implantable Doppler, which uses high-frequency ultrasound (20 MHz) with a 1 mm^2 crystal that can act as both transmitter and receiver for direct monitoring of the microvascular anastomosis.

A silicone cuff is placed around the vessel (**Figure 17.3**). The cuff is usually secured around the vessel with a small hemoclip. The wires exit the wound and are sutured to

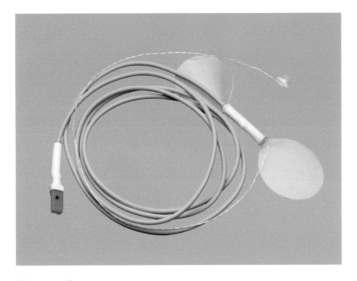

Figure 17.3 Silicone cuff.

the skin. The probe must be correctly placed during surgery since adjustments are not possible postoperatively.

The importance of early intervention to salvage flaps is well known. It is therefore critical to be able to assess and identify failing flaps early.

To date, no system has proved totally reliable. If there is any doubt at all about the patency of the anastomosis, it is best to reexplore a flap.

Microsurgical robotics

The Symani® Surgical System is a flexible platform consisting of two robotic arms that can be easily positioned to facilitate surgical procedures (**Figure 17.4**).

The system features 7–20× motion scaling with tremor filtration to address the demands and complexity of microsurgery and supermicrosurgery. Vessels less than 1 mm can be sutured. This is an ongoing field of development.

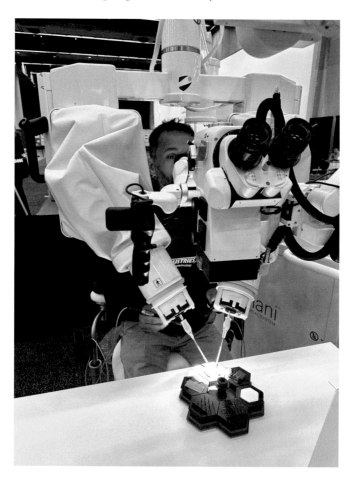

Figure 17.4 Prof. Ahmed suturing a 1 mm vessel.

Index

Note: Page numbers in *italics* refer to figures.

A

Acland clamps, 8–9, *8*, 56, 81, 82, 88, 91, 130, 132, 133
Anaesthetic management
    long-acting anaesthesia, 29–30
    rabbits, 30
    rats, 28–29
    short-acting anaesthesia, 29
Anastomosis with single clamps
    double clamp advantages, 96
    double *vs.* single clamps, 96
    one side up, 95, *95*
    single clamp disadvantages, 96
Anastomotic success
    alterations in blood flow, 34
    coagulation factors, 34
    coping mechanisms, 39
    failure of patency, 32
    gentle dissection, 32
    human factors, 38–39
    longitudinal torsion, 33, *33*
    mental efficiency, 38–39
    microsurgical technique faults, 32–33
    personal comfort, 38
    spasm, vessel musculature, 34–38
Animal model
    anaesthetic management, 28–30
    microsurgical skills, 28
    operating site preparation, 30
    pharmacological agents, 30–31
Animals Scientific Procedures Act, 28
Anticoagulant, 30
Arterial anastomosis
    Acland vessel, 44
    arterial clamping, *44*
    arterial clamp removal, 50–51, *51*
    arterial patency, 52
    clamp placement, *44*
    complete both stay stitches, 48, *49*
    heparinised saline, 44, 45
    irrigating the artery, 45, *45*
    milking test, 52
    needle placement, 46, 47, *47*
    one-way-up anastomosis, 52, *53*
    releasing tension, 50, *50*
    removing arterial adventitia, 46, *46*
    throw of stay stitch, 48, *48*
    venous anastomosis, 53–55, *54*, *55*
    venous patency, 55
    vessel dissection, 41–43
    vessel exposure, 40–41

C

Clinical practice
    anastomotic patency, 154, *154*
    intraoperative vessels, 150–151
    microsurgical instruments, 150
    operating microscope, 149
    patency tests, 154
    postoperative monitoring, 155–156
    preoperative procedures, 149
    setup for anastomoses, 151–152
    silicone cuff, 155, *155*
    suturing, 152–153
    vein grafts, 151
    vessel preparation, 152–153

E

End-to-end arterial anastomosis
    posterior wall exposure, 99, *99*
    remove distal clamp, 99, *100*
    single clamp application, 96, *97*
    single clamp 'weights,' 98, *98*
    stay sutures, 98, *98*
    triangulation technique, 97, *98*
End-to-end venous anastomosis
    anterior wall, 101, *101*
    posterior wall, 102, *102*
    remove proximal clamp, 103, *103*
    triangulation techniques, 101
End-to-side anastomosis
    anterior wall, 60–61, *61*
    carotid artery preparation, 64–66, *64–66*
    clamp removal, 62–63, *63*

femoral artery to carotid loop, 63
perform arteriotom, 59
perform venotomies, 58–59, *59*
posterior wall, 61–62, *62*
venotomy/arteriotomy length, 58
venotomy in rat model, *57*, 57–58
End-to-side continuous suturing
  anastomoses, 120
  aorta/vena cava vessel preparation, 118, *119*
  arterial anastomosis, *124*, 124–126, *125*
  clamp removal, 126, *126*
  renal exposure in rat, 116
  renal harvest, 116–118, *117–118*
  renal model, 115–116
  venous anastomosis, 120–123, *120–123*
Epigastric arterial anastomosis, 84–85, *85*
Epigastric artery and vein
  arterial cannulation, 83, *84*
  arterial dilatation, 82, *82*
  gentle massage of the artery, 81, *81*
  microvascular clamps, 81
  vein flushing, 83, *83*
  vessel irrigation, 82, *82*
Epigastric venous anastomosis, 86–87, *86–87*
Euthanasia, 31

F

Femoral artery anastomosis
  anterior wall into mouth, 106, *106*
  clamp removal, 108, *109*
  needle inside of anastomosis, 107, *107*
  stay suture detachment, 108, *108*
  stay suture placement, 105, *105*, 106, *106*
  vessels under 1 mm, 89–90, *89–90*
Femoral artery preparation, 88, *88*
Femoral vein anastomosis
  anterior wall, 91, *91*
  anterior wall stitch, 112, *113*
  clamp removal, 113, *113*
  double throw to stay stitch, 112, *112*
  flap reperfusion, 92, *93*
  needle inside of anastomosis, 111, *111*
  patency test, 92, *93*
  posterior wall, 91, *92*
  previous 'loop' as stay suture, 112, *113*
  renal vessels end-to-end continuous suturing, 114, *114*

  stay suture attachment, 110, *110*, *111*
  surface of the vein, 91

I

Interpositional vein graft
  anastomotic site, 70, *70*
  arterial anastomosis, 71, *71*
  clamp removal, 72–73, *73*
  discrepant-sized vein graft, 68, *69*
  distal anastomosis, 71–72, *72*
  epigastric vein graft, 67, *67*, 74–78, *74–78*
  femoral vein graft, 67, *67*
  120° to 120° suture placement, 70, *70*

M

Microscope
  care, 2–3
  eyepieces, 2
  illumination system, 2
  magnification, 1, 3
  objective lenses, 1
  optical system, 1–2, *2*
  optional, 1
  parts, *3*
  recommendations, 1
  setup, 3–4
  tiltable binocular tube, 2
Microsurgical instruments, *6*
  Acland clamps, 8–9, *8*
  adventitia scissors, 8
  care of instruments, 9–10
  dissecting scissors, 7–8
  features, 6
  hand position, 13–14, *14*
  jeweller/watchmaker forceps, 7
  needle holders, 7
  needles, 12
  Potts scissors, 8
  practice starter kit, 9, *10*
  rubber practice card, 13
  stitch formation, 14
  suture materials, 11, *11*
  tubal clamps, 9, *9*
  Vannas scissors, 8
  vessel dilator, 7
Microsurgical training models
  biological models, 27, *27*
  living model, 27

Penrose drain tubing, 25
silastic tubing, 25, *26*

P

Peripheral nerve repair, *127*
nerve model, 127
rat sciatic nerve, 128–134

R

Rat epididymovasostomy
advantages, 142–143
adventitia removal, 144, *144*
anatomy, 143, *143*
artery of vas deferens, 144, *144*
clamps, *142*
dissection, 143–148, *143–148*
dividing vas, 145, *145*
epididymis tubule, 146, *146*
incising caudal sac, 145, *145*
incising tubule transversely, 147, *147*
insert sutures, 147, *147*
monofilament nylon sutures, 146, *146*
secure vas muscularis, 148, *148*
vas lumen exposed, 146, *146*
Rat sciatic nerve
Acland clamp, 132, 133
anterior wall, 130, *131*
clamp repositioned, 132, *132*
epineural repair, 129–133
interfasicular repair, 134, *134*
interpositional nerve grafts, 133, *134*
nerve dissection, 129, *129*
nerve rotated, 132, *132*
posterior wall, 130, *131*
sciatic exposure, 128, *128*
stay suture placement, 130, *130*
tension release, 129, *129*
Rat vasovasostomy
advantages, 136
adventitia removal, 138, *138*
anatomy, 137, *137*
anterior wall, 140, *140*
artery of vas deferens, 138, *138*
clamps, *135*
posterior wall, 140, *140*
stitch last quadrant, 141, *141*
stitch placement, 139, *139*
two-layer method, 137
vas disection, 136, *136*
Respiratory stimulant, 31

S

Spasm, vessel musculature
affecting factors, 37
carotid artery, 34, *35*
discrepancy in vessel size, 35–37
flow, 37
repair, 38
Stitch formation
anterior wall, 21–22
assessment of suture lines, 22–23
hand position, 13–14, *14*
knot tying, 17–18, *17–19*
learning, 16
microsurgical instruments, 14
needle handling, 15, *15*
perfect stitch, 23–24, *24*
posterior wall, 22
procedures, *16*, 16–17
rubber glove exercise, 19–20
rubber practice card, 13
stay suture stitch, 21, *21*
triangulation technique, 20, *20*
Surgical loupes, *4*, 4–5
Suturing techniques
advantages, 104
anastomosis, 104
disadvantages, 104
femoral artery continuous anastomosis,
105–109, *105–109*
femoral vein continuous anastomosis,
109–113, *109–113*
reverse triangulation technique, 105

T

Tubal clamps, 9, *9*

V

Vasodilating agent, 31
Vessels under 1 mm
chicken model, 79
epigastric arterial anastomosis, 84–85, *85*
epigastric artery and vein, 80–84, *81–84*
epigastric venous anastomosis, 86–87,
86–87
femoral artery anastomosis, 89–90, *89–90*
femoral artery preparation, 88, *88*
femoral vein anastomosis, 91–93, *91–93*
rat and chicken models, 79
rat groin flap, *79*, 79–80, 94